Moments that Matter:
Cases in Ethical Eldercare

Jan 2011

To Marilyn,
Best wishes

[signature]

Previously Published Books

Old Enough to Feel Better: A Medical Guide for Seniors (1981, 1989)

An Ounce of Prevention: The Canadian Guide to a Healthy and Successful Retirement (1984)

Prévoir Les Belles Années De La Retraite (1986)

The Encyclopedia of Health and Aging (2001)

Parenting Your Parents: Support Strategies for Meeting the Challenge of Aging in the Family (2002, 2005)

Parenting Your Parents: Support Strategies for Meeting the Challenge of Aging in America (2006)

Brooklyn Beginnings: A Geriatrician's Odyssey (2009)

Moments that Matter: Cases in Ethical Eldercare

◆

A Guide for Family Members

Michael Gordon M.D., MSc, FRCPC

iUniverse, Inc.
New York   Bloomington

Moments that Matter: Cases in Ethical Eldercare
A Guide for Family Members

Copyright © 2010 by Michael Gordon M.D., MSc, FRCPC

All rights reserved. No part of this book may be used or reproduced by any means, graphic, electronic, or mechanical, including photocopying, recording, taping or by any information storage retrieval system without the written permission of the publisher except in the case of brief quotations embodied in critical articles and reviews.

The information, ideas, and suggestions in this book are not intended as a substitute for professional medical advice. Before following any suggestions contained in this book, you should consult your personal physician. Neither the author nor the publisher shall be liable or responsible for any loss or damage allegedly arising as a consequence of your use or application of any information or suggestions in this book.

iUniverse books may be ordered through booksellers or by contacting:

iUniverse
1663 Liberty Drive
Bloomington, IN 47403
www.iuniverse.com
1-800-Authors (1-800-288-4677)

Because of the dynamic nature of the Internet, any Web addresses or links contained in this book may have changed since publication and may no longer be valid. The views expressed in this work are solely those of the author and do not necessarily reflect the views of the publisher, and the publisher hereby disclaims any responsibility for them.

ISBN: 978-1-4502-0376-0 (sc)
ISBN: 978-1-4502-0378-4 (dj)
ISBN: 978-1-4502-0377-7 (ebk)

Library of Congress Control Number: 2010902210

Printed in the United States of America

iUniverse rev. date: 03/05/2010

*Dedicated to all my patients and their families who have
allowed me into their lives over all these years
and to my family, who have supported my efforts to fulfill my
dreams as a physician, teacher, and writer*

Contents

Introduction	xi
1. The Nature of Aging and the Health Care System	1
Myths about Aging	2
Using the Health Care System Well	4
2. You and Your Aging Family Member: Maintaining the Fabric of Caring and Love	6
3. Concepts of Medical Ethics, and How They Relate to Aging	12
Translating Ethical Concepts into Meaningful Action	12
The Meaning of Ethics in Everyday Terms	15
Narrative Ethics: A Place for "Me"	17
Maximizing Life or Extending It	19
Gulliver's Travels: Lessons to Be Learned?	23
The Timeline of Decline	25
Common, Everyday Activities: Driving	30
Romance and Sex	34
4. Decision-Making: The Individual and the Surrogate Decision Maker	42
Shifting the Balance	45
How Decisions Are Made: Personal and Ethical Aspects	46
Is There a Way to Make Things Clear?	47
5. Truth-Telling as an Example of Balancing Benefits and Harms	49
6. Challenges in Age-Based Medical Care: It Isn't Easy to Be Old and Sick	55
Why the Ageism?	56
Trying to Assure Good Care	58
7. Balancing Acts: When Goals Conflict	60

8. The Many Players in Ethics and Care	63
9. Is Quality of Life Everything? Secular and Religious Views	66
When ***Quality of Life*** Rather than Religious Issues Are in Question	71
10. Issues in Feeding and Drinking	78
The Meaning of Food and Drink	79
An Emotional Conflict with No Easy Answers	81
The Ethical Debate: Balancing the Principles	82
The Process of Decision-Making	83
When Feeding by Mouth Is the Right Choice—Even if Dangerous	86
Framing the Ethical and Emotional Challenge	89
11. Levels of Care: Finding a Balance Between Giving and Receiving Care	92
Exploring the Ethical Issues: Who Makes the Choices of Treatment, and Why	95
12. Challenges Posed by the Acute Hospital System	97
How to Say "Yes" to Treatments	98
How to Say "No" to Treatments	103
13. Cardiopulmonary Resuscitation (CPR): Reality and Myth	107
14. Long-Term Care	114
Who Decides If a Move to a Long-Term Care Facility Is Necessary or Preferred?	117
What If the Parent Rejects Help?	119
Who Decides Where?	121
What Are the Limits to Care?	123
15. End-of-Life Care Decisions	126
Living Wills: Not Always the Answer	128
Stopping Treatment: How and Who Decides?	131
16. Palliative Care: Achieving the Goals of Comfort and Dignity	136
17. Ethical Perspectives of Health Care Professionals	143
The Duty of Health Care Professionals to Be Vaccinated	145
Conflicts with Patients and Families	148

18. The Final Journey	150
Glossary of Commonly Used Ethical Terms	151
Resources	157
About the Author	171
Index	173

Introduction

This book is the culmination of my professional and personal challenges in the care of elders. I have written many articles and books on this subject. During the past few years, I have been spending more time in my practice and in my educational roles addressing ethical issues with family members, often of the patients I care for or in groups of families who come for educational sessions. The concept of ethical challenges convinced me to undertake this book.

I am an academic geriatrician. I have been involved in the care of elders for more than thirty years as a clinician, educator, and administrator. I have learned a great deal through my professional roles. Dealing with the trials and tribulations of my own family has been just as important in understanding the challenges in eldercare. The melding of professional and personal experiences has helped me understand the challenges faced by families of aging individuals.

The stories in this book incorporate this interweaving of experiences. They are based on cases formulated in a way to protect the identity and privacy of those involved and are often a composite of similar cases. Names used are not real.

During the formative years of my life, I lived with my maternal grandmother, parents, and sister in a one-bedroom apartment in Brooklyn. Long before I even thought about medicine as a career, I had learned to cherish the devotion and stories of my grandmother, an immigrant from Lithuania. The last illness of her life had a profound influence on me even before I could understand the implications of the medical care she received at that time. Care options were fewer then, and my parents had to make critical decisions during the last few weeks of her life. Many years later, long after I was a mature and experienced physician, I had to face comparable decisions with my mother's final illness and death, and my father's gradual decline in function and increase in care needs.

My mother became ill in Brooklyn, which was our home during our developmental years, but no longer so. Many years before, I had moved to Toronto, and my sister, Diane (nicknamed Diti), had moved to Chicago. The months of our mother's illness were made more difficult by the need to travel back and forth to provide the care, support, and decision-making that my father needed and to be there when the difficult decisions that determined her future and care had to be made.

The experience with my mother highlighted the various conflicts and complex choices and conundrums family members face when difficult clinical and ethical decisions have to be made. With our father, who eventually agreed to move closer to my sister in Chicago as his own function declined, we became aware of the enormous challenges involved in making the best choices possible when it came to difficult medical care and personal decisions. Those personal experiences combined with the many ethically intriguing situations that I face in my professional medical role as a geriatrician and clinical ethicist have helped me explain to family members and health care professionals how to approach and help resolve the difficult challenges older people face—especially when they are ill or nearing the end of life.

This book is designed to help those like yourself who are charged with the responsibility of helping to make difficult decisions and to find the means to come to conclusions that satisfy the values and beliefs of those involved in receiving and providing care. Through reading the case-based analysis of common scenarios that reflect the struggles and triumphs of those involved in care decisions, you and other members of your family will be better equipped to help yourselves and your loved ones make the right decisions—ones with which you can live and look back on with a sense of accomplishment and peace.

The process of working through difficult decisions and weighing potentially conflicting choices can lead to an acceptable resolution. This process, when successful, should allow you and members of your family to go on with your lives and have a sense that what you did for your loved one was meaningful and enhanced the humanity and closeness in your own life and family relationships.

After some introductory chapters, which I hope will help focus your attention on the issues involved in decision-making with and for loved ones, case histories will highlight the important challenges that all of us face when helping to care for our aging parents or other elderly friends and family members. I will focus primarily on the ethical challenges that occur, which always include the relationships among you and other family members, no matter how close or estranged.

I start with some of the earlier challenges that may occur between elders and their children, which may not appear as dramatic as end-of-life decisions. These are often among the first challenges to arise when the weight of decision-making is partially if not fully transferred from the elder to you and other members of your family.

As the book progresses, I will address the more complex issues that occur over time and with which you and your family might struggle and for which you might seek ethical advice in addition to clinical information to help inform your final decisions. A glossary of commonly used ethical terms is included in the book to assist you and your family members in understanding the context and meaning of some of the discussions that might take place between you and members of the health care team who might be involved in carrying out decisions and care.

I wish to thank my wife, Gilda Berger, who encouraged me to write this book. Thanks to all of my patients, their families, my colleagues, medical trainees, and students and staff at Baycrest Geriatric Health Care System and the University of Toronto Joint Centre for Bioethics for all the support, insights, and help that they have provided over the past thirty-three years. In particular, I thank Mary McDiarmid of the Baycrest Library and Leslie Iancovitz from Baycrest's Department of Social Work, Wendy Harris of Johns Hopkins University Press, and Anne Miller, an associate in the world of writing, for valuable insights and comments on the structure and content of the book. I would also like to thank Dr. Muriel R. Gillick, Clinical Professor of Population Medicine at Harvard Medical School and Professor Steven R. Sabat, Ph.D., Professor of Psychology, Georgetown University for their invaluable comments and suggestions.

1

The Nature of Aging and the Health Care System

One of the great success stories of the last and present centuries is that more people are living into old age than ever before. The population in the Western world is aging rapidly. For many, the later years are full of satisfaction, with joys coming from watching families grow as well as from the pursuit of personal interests and activities. In response to the aging of the population, new opportunities have developed that did not exist years ago: special travel arrangements for seniors so they can continue to explore the world; educational opportunities at universities, colleges, and community centers that cater to all levels of curiosity and taste; and exercise and sports programs geared to those in the later years so they can develop and maintain physical prowess and function. New industries have grown to respond to the special interests and needs of the aging population.

But with all the successes, the reality for many older individuals is that at some time they may face a serious illness or decline in physical and mental function. The likelihood of developing certain types of ailments increases with age, even among those who take health promotion and disease prevention strategies seriously.

Although two-thirds of seniors may continue through their very late years with intact mental function, Alzheimer's disease and other causes of dementia may affect as many as one-third of people over the age of eighty-five. Other disorders that affect the heart, blood vessels, kidneys, and brain may be disabling. Care for those affected by diseases that undermine the ability to make decisions or provide self-care is being assumed by devoted sons and daughters like yourself and other members of your family.

Most families undertake the care of a loved one with enormous devotion and dedication. In a modern and busy world, it is often a mammoth challenge for families or sometimes friends to figure out who will do what and when for an ailing older parent, uncle, aunt, spouse, or significant other. Families and friends often come together to care for an older loved one, even at great personal, emotional, and financial stress. In a society in which families often live far from where they were born or where their loved ones reside, it is a greater challenge to meet some of the needs that may occur during times of crisis and physical or mental decline.

The concepts of medical ethics have entered mainstream medical care at these critical times, and, when faced with sensitive, threatening, and sometimes agonizing choices, you and your family may seek guidance as to the right or best way to make tough caregiving decisions. The ethical framework of such decision-making draws on many of the intrinsic values held by those of you involved in the decision-making process. These decisions are often affected by the ethical, religious, ethnic, cultural, and professional backgrounds of those of you involved. The values and beliefs of your parent who is usually the patient, of you and your family, and of professional caregivers must be taken into account. Also the cultural values and legal frameworks that exist in the community in which you all live become part of the consideration when decisions have to be made.

The media often present the aging of the population as a crisis because of the projected increased demands on health care and social service systems in addition to the increased involvement and responsibility of family members like you. But it is not beyond the capabilities of Western societies to respond in a positive and supportive manner to the existing and potential wishes and needs of the aging population. For the general population and those who are elected or appointed to develop public policy to properly fulfill the population's expectations of good-quality health care for the aging population, many myths about aging have to be dispelled.

Myths about Aging

One overarching myth is that every aged person will decline in health and function and therefore become a burden on his or her family and on the health care and social service systems. This includes the notion that these inevitable events will become a drain on valuable resources from other members of society, including the younger generation. A number of studies attest to the fact that the vast majority of older people continue to be productive members of society well into their very late years. Many work or volunteer as well as spend their money on household and other items, thereby contributing to the viability of society. Many not only contribute to their family's well-being through financial transfers from the older to the younger generation but also participate in child care for family members. No less important, many seniors act as mentors and role models to younger family members. Educators in the field of aging observe that many doctors who chose geriatrics and the care of elderly as a career path attribute their choice at least partly to the role modeling and closeness they experienced with older family members during their formative and critical developmental years.

Older individuals in your family and you with other members of your family can undertake many strategies to assure the best use of the health care system to fulfill your individual needs and reflect the best ethical values as to how all of us should use the available societal resources. One example is taking all steps possible to maximize your own health status.

Another myth about aging is that, after a certain time, which is never clearly defined, it is too late to make any health care changes that affect your future health or function. At any time of life, any of us at any age can make many changes in lifestyle that can result in physical or mental benefits to well-being and function. Whatever personal belief systems you have, you can make a good decision to maximize your health—whenever possible and within the limits of human disposition and frailty—through whatever lifestyle modifications that have been shown to have a positive effect on short-term and long-term health outcomes.

Most people, for example, know that cigarette smoking is not healthy. It is generally acknowledged that public health measures to decrease the likelihood of youngsters beginning to smoke, to decrease access to smoking venues, and to acknowledge the negative health aspects of secondhand smoke may decrease the need for health care resources for illnesses caused by smoking. Health care providers recognize how difficult it is for smokers to stop smoking even when they know about its negative health effects. Individuals can take some control of the decision-making process to stop smoking by exploring avenues that might work for them. Maybe it's through counseling sessions alone or in groups or the various medications developed to support those who have decided to stop smoking. Strong public policy supporting smoking bans and decreasing exposure to secondhand smoke (in restaurants, bars, airplanes, and public buildings, for example) has been shown to promote a culture of lower cigarette sales and less tobacco use.

Each of us can decrease our personal risk of needing the health care system for tobacco-related diseases (such as lung cancer, chronic bronchitis and emphysema, and heart disease) by taking on the improvement of our own health status and promoting and supporting public policy that does so at a societal level. For elders in your family who smoke, cessation can have sustained beneficial effects, and it is never too late to stop. Although the risk factor for lung cancer may not diminish substantially, because it is based on the cumulative effect of the previous years of tobacco exposure, effects on chronic lung and heart disease can be beneficial. There can be a decrease in susceptibility to lung infections and angina attacks with a discontinuation of smoking while the other medically necessary steps are taken. In addition to improving symptoms, if done properly, stopping smoking can demonstrate to an older family member that he or she can exercise some control over personal well-being. This often requires a concerted effort, which might include medications and group supports, which have become more available for those who wish to stop smoking. Also, grandparents can be instrumental in avoiding exposing grandchildren to secondhand smoke and not providing them with a negative role model. Resources to help in the process can be found at the Web sites of the American Lung Association and the Canadian Lung Association.

The same principles apply to many other aspects of health care for which preventive steps can supplement and perhaps decrease the need for formal health care–related treatments, such as surgery or medications for lifestyle-related illnesses. Personal lifestyle changes can decrease dependency on the health care system and its myriad treatments in a number of areas. These include obesity, a sedentary lifestyle, dietary choices that increase vascular (blood vessel) illnesses (such as blood pressure, heart attack, and stroke), and excessive use of potentially harmful agents such as alcohol and unnecessary prescription and over-the-counter medications.

It is a myth that older people can't exercise. Many senior programs have modified exercise programs for seniors, including those with physical disabilities. There are group programs for movement often with music, pool programs for those with arthritis or Parkinson's disease for which the buoyancy in water makes movements easier, and chair-based exercises for those who have decreased mobility. Many community-based senior programs cater to the older frail population, and these can usually be found through a community resource center. Many YMCAs and other such organizations have programs developed for and directed to the senior population.

Using the Health Care System Well

At some time, all of us will have to use some aspect of the formal health care system because of an illness or potentially disabling condition. The most important step any of us and our family members can take to assure the best outcomes possible is to know about the medical conditions being treated and what alternative and reasonable treatment options exist. Many individuals feel overwhelmed by the health care system and the number of health care professionals with whom they must communicate. Sometimes patients and their families do not ask reasonable and important questions for fear of appearing foolish or to avoid conflict with health care providers. But asking reasonable and well-thought-out questions should result in a reasoned response.

In 2007, in its quest to decrease untoward or adverse outcomes among older hospitalized patients in the United States and enhance overall quality of care, Medicare, the primary insurer for older Americans, indicated that it would not reimburse hospitals for certain adverse outcomes that were avoidable, thus putting the onus on hospitals and health care providers to take steps to provide optimal care to their patients. The patients would not be responsible for the payments; rather, the potential loss of reimbursement to the hospitals is believed to be a motivating force to improve the quality of hospitalizations and care.

Points to Remember

- There are many myths about aging—one of which is that all elders become increasingly frail and ultimately dependent.
- People age at varying rates, depending on biological and environmental factors.
- Each of us can make some lifestyle changes to decrease the rate and degree of functional decline and thereby maximize function and active participation in life.
- If you must use the health care system, be knowledgeable about the medical conditions being treated and ask about what alternative and reasonable treatment options exist.

2

You and Your Aging Family Member: Maintaining the Fabric of Caring and Love

Your family structure and the relationships among its members is probably one of the most important aspects of life. During our developmental years, a major part of our human endeavor is focused on how we grow and relate to our parents, grandparents, and siblings. In later life, it is how we relate to a spouse, children, grandchildren, and extended family. The old adage "blood is thicker than water" reflects the almost-universal acknowledgment that the way we connect to our family, even those who may be distant, is special.

Even though many of us have friends with whom we might share more of our daily lives, family ties matter to a great degree to most of us. These bonds often become more important during the later years.

Unfortunately, it is common for family ties to become stretched and challenged when families face the decline of a parent. This is especially true when it appears that one member of the family is carrying an inordinate amount of the care responsibilities.

I recently experienced a situation in which a son of an elderly woman who had significant dementia turned up for the first time in my office accompanying his mother. His father was being strained beyond his coping abilities but would not consider any external assistance, community program, or institutional care. Also at the visit was his younger sister, with whom I had worked over the previous year and who was the primary caregiver for their parents, who were clearly struggling to maintain themselves in the community.

The son became involved when he recognized that a crisis was brewing. Somehow he erroneously assumed that his sister was not being forceful enough to get things done or did not know what she was doing; therefore, he thought he had to, in his own words, "make things happen."

The burning question to be considered was how did this family address the family and ethical issue of who was going to make decisions for the parents. The mother clearly was not in a position to make significant decisions about her care because of her mental incapacity. Was her husband able to do so? The daughter had always carried the responsibility of working through the family dynamics; her father had the notion that everything would be okay and refused to acknowledge the stress he was under and the negative effect his indecision had on his daughter. The daughter's personal life and family were stressed by the demands being made on her time and physical and emotional energy.

Until the visit to my office, the son, who was being protected by his father and sister because, as they said repeatedly, "He is too busy with his company," was only tangentially engaged. When he came to the visit, perhaps as a way to justify his absence for most of the time, he emphasized how busy he was, how many hours he worked, and how many people he employed.

Now the son was going to take charge (as he did with his business) and wanted answers and clear direction, which, as he learned, was easier asked for than done. He said he would make sure his father listened to him about his mother's needs. He seemed to overlook or diminish the fact that his sister was undertaking most of the arrangements and would run to their parents' home in the middle of the night when the mother was wandering about the house. He was not aware that his mother would at times begin to bake cakes in the kitchen for a holiday that was not occurring and reject her husband's pleas to return to bed.

With some discussion, the son began to appreciate the complexity of what was going on and how a "quick fix" was not possible. Suggestions were made as to social work assistance and the need to make plans and consider future options for care. Because it appeared that the mother was not capable of making decisions for herself, the immediate ethical issues were these:

- Who could not just legally but actually make the choices for the mother?
- When choices were considered on behalf of the mother, what if those choices had a serious negative effect on the patient and the other family members?
- What if the father/husband refused any external help, even though it put his wife at some risk of injury?
- What if the son made certain decisions on behalf of his parents that his sister thought were potentially dangerous?

- What if the son wanted to do things that were in conflict with the parents' wishes and desires?
- What could or should the daughter do to try to achieve positive goals while at the same time avoiding harming her parents' interests and avoiding major conflict with her older brother?

Families often do not think of the decisions that they make within a formal ethical framework; rather, decision-making is based on the relationships and values they share and their varied abilities and interests. It is unfortunate when sometimes complex and difficult family dynamics and ethical principles are not considered when difficult care decisions are contemplated. At the extreme, some families resort to the legal route to solve such problems, which is most unfortunate. On rare occasions, I have seen families in which siblings communicated only through third parties (sometimes another sibling) or lawyers to provide necessary care because of a fracture in their relationship that could not be overcome when a crisis loomed.

Using ethical frameworks in addition to the natural sense of love and kinship can assist in resolving some of the tensions that often exist even within highly cohesive families and can facilitate reaching a common ground in the decision-making process. For example, in the case just described, the son and daughter could take the opportunity to try together as loving children and siblings to decipher the ethical challenges and issues that face their father and mother. They could ultimately acknowledge that their father wants to do the right and best thing for his wife.

The issue then becomes whether or not their father is capable of representing their mother, who clearly cannot manifest her own will because of severe dementia. Can their father reasonably reflect her autonomous choices or best interests as the surrogate decision maker? The use of a surrogate decision maker is the legal way of translating the ethics principle of autonomy into a legally understood action. If their father can represent his wife's wishes in a reasonably honest fashion because of the many years that he has known her and lived with her, that is his responsibility. This is so even if his children disagree with his decisions. They must respect his ethical and legal responsibility to do so. It may come to be that the only step they can take at this point is to assist him as he struggles to achieve his goals, even at the risk of failure.

The two siblings should try to clarify between themselves and with their father how decision-making will be undertaken if and when their father is not able to make decisions on behalf of their mother (and maybe on his own behalf). To respect as much as possible their parents' personal choices and preferences, they should try to explore what kinds of decisions might be considered acceptable in difficult clinical situations or in the most challenging end-of-life situations. If, for example, their parents were devoutly Catholic, do the children think that the parents would want religious considerations to come into play if a tube feeding or a respirator was necessary? How would they feel about asking a priest for advice on whether or not to discontinue treatment that did not seem likely to be successful? Combining their love and devotion for their parents with a mutually agreeable ethical framework in which the benefits and avoidance of risks or harms are taken into account can help the children review what issues should be considered when such difficult decisions have to be made.

There are no easy solutions to complex family situations. Sometimes for family peace, family members may defer to those who have apparently preferential positions in the family rather than contradict those who feel responsible for making the important decisions. A combination of family dynamics, family history, and cultural practice may determine who will ultimately make the most difficult decisions.

During a recent case of mine dealing with end-of-life care for a retired university professor who had severe dementia, his wife was certain that, in addition to refusing a feeding tube, which she had previously discussed with him on a number of occasions, he would not want to have his life prolonged by the use of intravenous or subcutaneous (under the skin) fluids. A physician son, who was living abroad and had not been involved in any of the day-to-day struggles with his father's progressive dementia but who was a supportive and loving child, could not accept the withdrawal of fluid replacement for his father. But, in the name of family peace, the physician son's views swayed his mother, who legally was the surrogate but could not bring herself to go against her son, whose motivation she respected.

The wife admitted to me that her husband, in addition to having expressed his views on such treatment, might also have acceded to his son's instructions as part of his desire to always support the concept of family peace. If giving fluids would make them feel that they had done everything and be better able to live with themselves after his death, the wife conceded that the professor might not have objected to the extension of his life by two weeks, which turned out to be the case. At the end, the family seemed to be cohesive in their belief that they did everything possible to meet his needs for comfort and had acted as benevolently as any family could under the circumstances.

I was speaking at one of many public presentations to children of aging parents. The audience consisted of fifteen female, mostly middle-aged employees. As the presentation progressed, it was clear from the audience reaction that many of my topics resonated strongly among them. The topic of getting a proper geriatric assessment and the issue of guilt and its position in the equation of feelings that are shared among parents and their children were clearly of great concern. Many in the audience acknowledged that feelings of guilt were pervasive. There seemed to be a challenge in what to do with guilt feelings and whether they promoted or interfered with the relationship with the aging parent or ultimately resulted in better care despite the uneasy feelings related to this deep-seated emotion.

From the feelings of guilt felt by many members of the audience there seemed to develop among some a concern about how and what to communicate to one's loved ones. Sometimes, even among a group of devoted children and a household that was close, communication about important or emotionally laden issues was not common. The reality is that without open and frank communication, little of importance can be achieved.

Within the contemporary framework of ethics, the concept of respect for autonomy requires that people be involved in decision-making that affects their lives. Most children want to respect that attribute, but may be afraid to confront sensitive issues or be misinterpreted as wanting to make decisions or take over a parent's decision-making role. This might be perceived or expressed even while the parent wants the children's help to cope with the difficult decisions that have to be faced. The challenges may also be different if you are an only child or if you no longer live geographically close to your parent or parents.

Toward the end of the talk, during the interactive part of the program, a member of the audience, an only child, recounted a recent experience of arranging for an in-home geriatric assessment in the face of objections by her parents, who lived far from where she lived and worked. What drove her determination to seek the assessment was the fact that she could not provide the kind of care that she believed her parents, both still living in their home, needed to remain there. The daughter spoke about her feelings of guilt with the knowledge that she had chosen to work in a place that was far away for good career and personal family reasons even though it would likely present difficulties. She was racked by the guilt of not fulfilling her duties as a loving daughter even though she recognized her parents' strong sense of independence and privacy. Because of these feelings, they had previously rejected any in-home geriatric assessment and expressed to her strongly that it was not necessary, and they were fine.

Then came the mother's fall that resulted in a fractured wrist. The effect on her independence and her husband's ability to look after her was substantial. She needed help in dressing, toileting, and bathing. Her husband realized that he could not attend to her needs, especially those that normally required substantial physical effort and a level of personal and private intervention (such as toileting). Fortunately, on relatively short notice, the local community care service provider (also often known as a home care agency) was able to provide some in-home assistance and that, coupled with some private daily help, allowed the couple to cope during the eight-week period before a semblance of independence could be regained. But the involvement of the agency and its workers promoted the daughter's ability to arrange for a geriatric assessment, which her parents now welcomed despite some pride and privacy-driven reluctance.

The daughter recounted what a beneficial effect the assessment had, not only on home safety changes but also on how some daily tasks, such as shopping and cooking, were restructured. Most important, after the interaction and changes were implemented, the father acknowledged that the input from the "team," especially the assessment nurse, was "really good." He went on to welcome future suggestions and care plans now that he understood how they would enhance his and his wife's safety and their ability to remain in their home. The daughter acknowledged that it was going to be a long struggle, but with a formalized and structured program in place, her guilt was partially assuaged. She felt it deeply when trying to help her parents before events resulted ultimately in the necessity of their agreement to receive help. Guilt had led to a positive result, which is the most favorable outcome of that powerful emotion.

Points to Remember

- Most of you and your family want to do the best for your aging parents.
- Even in the face of family disharmony and a history of discord, many families can find ways to come together during critical times to help an elderly loved one cope with the challenges of physical and mental decline.
- The key to helping aging parents is to have the necessary conversations to understand their values and how to help them achieve their goals.
- The process of getting to where you want to be as a loving child or other family member may be long and arduous, but it is important to persevere, knowing that there may be failures along the way before there are any successes.

3

Concepts of Medical Ethics, and How They Relate to Aging

Translating Ethical Concepts into Meaningful Action

With the importance of the family fabric acknowledged as the key to all family relationships and ultimately to much if not all decision-making, it is important to understand some of the definitions and meanings of ethics when it comes to decision-making.

We all want the best for our parents. Sometimes it is hard to know what the best is, and if not all of the choices are good, we hope that one of the choices is clearly better than the other ones. Health and well-being and the absence of disease or the ability to withstand the onslaught of illness can be a complex and daunting affair for your aging parent and you and other members of your family. Those of us who have raised children know the anguish we feel when a child is ill. Physicians and other health care providers are usually aware of the anxiety that parents feel in the face of a child's illness, even one that appears to be fairly simple and innocuous.

I recall when my youngest child had a ruptured appendix at age six. My wife and I were devastated that he could be so ill, especially when early on we were led to believe that he had a simple gastrointestinal viral infection. The subsequent terrible pain and the urgent surgery and the complicated postoperative course, his delirium and then his slow recovery and urgent readmission for a wound abscess challenged us as loving parents. With an aging parent, the emotional strains can be as intense, although the terror may not be as severe as with a child because of the more natural order of the expectations that exist for the later stages in life.

Wanting the best outcome is therefore a natural feeling that you will have as an adult child when your aging parent becomes ill. When the process is gradual, as often occurs with diseases of later years such as dementia of the

Alzheimer's type, you may get used to and become knowledgeable of the process. But that does not protect you from the realities of the often difficult choices to be made. That is where an understanding of ethics and "doing the right thing" becomes important to you and members of your family.

Let us imagine that you are a loving daughter watching your mother suffering and dying from incurable cancer. All the treatments available have been tried. Some novel treatments are offered in other parts of the world, but they would not be covered by any health care system, and you do not have the money to pay for them. You wonder if it is fair that the government or your insurance company won't pay because, after all, your mother's life is at risk. On the other hand, you can understand that there have to be some limits on how money is spent for health care in general. You are torn between your personal wishes and needs and your recognition of a mutual obligation to use fairly the resources we all share.

You have come to terms with the fact that insurance will not pay for going to Mexico for an unproven treatment and your mother's suffering is increasing despite reasonable attempts at palliative care. One day, she says, "Can't you do something to help end this suffering quickly? I have had enough. Please help me. Give me something."

You are terrified. You cannot imagine doing something like that to your mother, but she is suffering. You speak to the wonderful nurse who has been looking after her in the hospital. The bed in the hospice has been applied for but will not be available for another week. They have been giving advice to the staff at the general hospital for pain management, but when your mother gets what she needs, she seems to become confused and drowsy, and that is hard for you to witness.

You speak to the nurse: "My mother asked me to help end her life. I know that is something that I cannot do. Can she not be given something to make it go faster?"

The nurse has heard it before and says, "You know that professionally and ethically we cannot hasten her death. Speak to the doctor about changing her pain medication. Maybe she can come up with something that will help you and your mother."

You are emotionally torn because you want to help your mother, but you know that you cannot ask the doctor to do something unprofessional, unethical, and illegal. You approach the doctor and explain your dilemma.

The doctor explains the situation from the professional and medically ethical perspective: "I cannot give your mother anything for the specific purpose of ending her life. In some parts of the world, such as the Netherlands and even in Oregon or the state of Washington in the United States, there are methods that might allow a physician to assist in hastening death or provide an individual with the means that they can use themselves, but those practices are not legal in Canada or other parts of the United States. Moreover, even if they were, I would not be able to participate for my own professional and ethical reasons."

Your heart sinks as you realize that you might not be able to help your mother's suffering even though you understand and at some level agree with what the doctor is telling you.

The doctor continues, "We can help your mother's suffering and discomfort from her malignant pain, but the outcome has to be acceptable to you and to her. First of all, if we use sufficient pain medication in the right combinations, we can usually decrease or eliminate the most terrible of her pain. However, she may be less responsive and even more likely to be sleepy and lethargic. In some cases, with such a pain management process, it was previously believed that life expectancy might be marginally shortened, but this does not seem to be the case in most instances. The goal of treatment is to relieve suffering and with the right medication combinations this is usually possible."

You ask the doctor, "If she dies sooner than she might have otherwise died, is that not the same as killing her?"

The doctor's reply is comforting: "First of all this is not usually the case if the medications are used properly with gradual increases in doses as required for symptom relief. Secondly, as long as the intention is to treat her pain and make her comfortable and relieve her suffering, the fact that her death may occur somewhat earlier than if we had not tried to relieve her unbearable suffering does not mean we are committing an act of euthanasia. The intent is what matters, and for us the intent is to treat her pain effectively and adequately. As long as we all understand what we are doing and accept the consequences of good pain and symptom management, we are acting ethically, professionally, and legally."

If you agreed and gave the doctor permission to carry on, it is likely that within a few days to a week there would be a decrease in your mother's pain. As it happened in this case, it became obvious to all concerned because there was less crying out and grimacing, but this was coupled with fewer moments of full wakefulness. When the end came, which was anticipated and planned for, it was clear from the daughter's feelings and comments that the "right" thing had been done and the proper tenets of ethically sound care were adhered to for the sake of a suffering patient and her loving family.

The Meaning of Ethics in Everyday Terms

For most people, ethics means "doing the right or best thing." We often think of words like *morality* and sometimes mix up the ideas of ethics with the concepts of law. Most people think of themselves as ethical and are often disturbed when they recognize that something has happened that they perceive as wrong but don't know what to do with it. Many parents when raising children try to instill in them a sense of ethics and frame the concepts in terms that make good sense.

Our ethical principles in everyday life come from countless sources. For many of you, a religious source may be the basis of your belief system, even if you are not particularly observant in that religion. The prohibitions and expectations of the major religions have had a major effect on many of our societal values, which are often translated into our laws.

In an ideal world, we hope that our laws would reflect good and universally acceptable ethical principles. Yet we know that sometimes the law seems to be out of step with important ethical tenets, although it may be that for some the law reflects their ethical principle and for others the law conflicts with it. Examples are the laws that over the years have dealt with contentious issues such as abortion and euthanasia. In different parts of the world, the practices and the corresponding laws are different, which suggests that some issues may not be universally accepted as core ethical values for a given society or for some people in any society, whatever laws exist.

In the end-of-life dilemma noted in the case just described, the ethical principles that are often referred to in North America include concepts such as *autonomy*, which means respecting the wishes of the person (the patient usually) when under medical care. If the patient is not able to make decisions about his or her own health care needs, it is often necessary for a family member to take on the role and act on the person's behalf as was the situation in this case where the daughter ended up having to make the difficult decisions regarding palliative care and pain management. The idea and ethical principle of *beneficence* is what motivates most people who choose to be doctors and nurses—that is, the commitment to help people and relieve suffering. Of course, family members are usually motivated by the same impulses, but not as part of their professional role. When the doctor suggested a regimen of pain management to relieve the otherwise resistant pain, *beneficence* was being expressed.

Another important ethical principle that is the focus of ethical decision-making is the notion of *nonmaleficence,* which is the avoidance of unnecessary harm. Going as far back as the ancient Greek physician Hippocrates, the notion of the duty to avoid causing harm has been paramount in the professional ethics of physicians and should be considered as important to family members. In the case of the mother's pain, we could consider which harm was worse: that of uncontrollable pain or a somewhat premature but inevitable death. Considering the circumstances of this scenario, the professional staff and ultimately the family believed that the pain was causing the far greater harm; therefore, they agreed to pain management even at the potential risk of perhaps an earlier death or more likely, a greater degree of lassitude.

The last of the main ethical principles is called *justice,* meaning distributive justice or, as most people would think of it, fairness. It is the process by which we collectively decide what is the fairest way to provide the care to all of those in need of care considering all the other people and with the resources that we have available to us.

In the previous example, if the daughter had asked that the nurse for the unit spend all of her time with her mother because "she was dying," that would have meant that none of the other patients on the unit might have received the care they needed and also deserved. If the daughter insisted that a certain pain medication, which was perhaps marginally better but would not significantly affect the treatment outcome of her mother, be used even though it was ten times the cost of the standard treatment, we could question the ethics of using such limited resources in such a manner.

Such questions come up every day in the world of contemporary health care: Which drug for which person? Who gets into an intensive care unit bed? How does one adjust the list for urgent surgery? Who decides on what treatments are available to which members of society when there isn't enough money or resources to treat everyone for everything?

These are the basic concepts or as we call them *principles of contemporary medical ethics.* You and your family may need help in the difficult decision-making processes. It becomes important to try to understand the concepts around these principles so that when you are called on to exercise your roles in caring for your loved ones; you can help make the best decisions possible and do the right thing within an understandable and agreed-to framework.

Points to Remember

- Examining how children make complex decisions about their parents' care will often reveal that there is an ethical component to all important decisions that are made.
- It can be useful for family members to understand and appreciate the ethics context in which such difficult decisions are made.

- All families struggle with difficult decisions for their aging family members. Family dynamics, family history, and other factors will always interface with ethical principles in the decision-making process.
- The recognition of the ethical component of decision-making can be helpful to children of aging parents as most, no matter what else may be going on, want to "do the right thing" when it comes to difficult late-life decisions.

Narrative Ethics: A Place for "Me"

In the past few years, partially in reaction to what is often called the *principlist* approach to ethics in which the focus of ethical decision-making is on the four principles mentioned previously (autonomy, beneficence, nonmaleficence, and justice), the focus on the individual's narrative or story has developed. This has been a countervailing force to balance some of the observed deficiencies in *principlism* as the commonly used approach to ethical decision-making.

The essence of narrative ethics is that by delving into the person's "story," meanings may come forth that may give a greater insight and understanding than a focus on the standard ethical principles might provide.

An example of a case I was involved with some years ago should help illustrate this concept. Mrs. F was 86 years old and had been a patient of mine for almost five years while she lived in a retirement home attached to the geriatric complex in which I worked. I was requested to see her because she had refused an offer of dialysis for chronic renal failure. "I'm old and have no one left in the world that is close to me. What reason is there to live?" This is what she said to me when I asked her why she had declined dialysis. She was a Polish immigrant, widow, and childless, as the children she had from her first marriage perished in the Holocaust. Without dialysis she would die.

She continued with her explanation, "You know that I lost all of my family in the Holocaust. I had a husband and two children who were eight and five at the time that they were taken from me. I remarried after the war to a Canadian man who came from a town near my own in Poland, but before the war. We did not have any children, and he died more than 12 years ago. I have been alone ever since. I worked as a seamstress but could not continue because of poor vision, and within five years of his death I stopped working, living on a modest pension from his work and some reparations from Germany. The only person left is a distant cousin who lives in Ottawa, Ontario, whom I haven't seen in four years, and she is quite ill herself."

As Mrs. F revealed more personal reflections about her own values, beliefs, and memories, woven into a fairly coherent narrative spanning several decades, there was a special space opened between us, and a different kind of knowing, for both of us, became possible. She was not simply a "patient with renal failure" but a person with layers of stories, memories, and meaningful experiences important for me to know something about.

The nurses and the attending physician had referred Mrs. F. to me to see if I could "convince" her to agree to dialysis, as I had known her since the time she moved into the retirement home. It was I who had referred her to the nephrologists some years before. After a psychiatric consultation, which refuted a diagnosis of possible depression, the feeling was that she was mentally capable of making her decision to forgo dialysis. She understood the potential benefits of treatment and the implications of refusal. I did my best to understand Mrs. F.'s life story and why she would refuse what was likely to be a life-saving treatment. I began as we spoke to understand her deep loneliness and sense of loss and absence of meaning to her life with no real connections of importance.

When Mrs. F asked me, "What is there to live for?" I responded while alone with her in her hospital room: "For me." She looked at me quizzically and asked, "Why for you?" I replied, "I want you to live longer because I like you and because I think the world will be less rich a place without you." She sat up more in bed and said, "Really?" in her strong Polish/Yiddish accent. "Is that really so?" My reply was, "Yes. I have always enjoyed seeing you at the retirement home's clinic and hearing from you about your experiences." She had recounted many stories of her life in her native Poland and her Holocaust experience, and how she had overcome the challenges when she arrived in Canada in her mid-30s.

She told me with pride how she struggled with English, found work, became involved in a group of like-minded friends, rebuilt her life with her second husband who then died, and how many of her friends were now old and frail like herself or had died. She became a volunteer and loved helping disabled children and that had become the focus of her life before she moved into the retirement home when even that activity had become too much for her. She looked at me and said, "You are a very nice doctor, and I would like to do this if it matters to you. But what if I am not happy with the treatment?" I replied, "If after three months of dialysis, you are not happy, we will stop it and make sure that your final days are as peaceful and comfortable as possible." She replied, "I will give it a try." The dialysis was successful and only after four years did she decide that it had become too much of a burden and we together with her nephrologist decided to discontinue the treatment and allow her to die peacefully.

This is an example of where if the standard ethical principle of autonomy would have been allowed to determine the course of her care, her initial refusal of the proposed treatment within a context of apparent cognitive competence would have resulted in her death four years previously. It was the pursuit of her "story" and what was meaningful in her life—that is relationships that allowed her to try the treatment which proved to be effective and acceptable to her for a period of four years. Her narrative allowed me to find the entrance of meaning into her life.

Maximizing Life or Extending It

It has become popular to talk or write about life extension as one of the options that the aging population has if they would take some specific actions, take some potions and pills, or often undertake a combination of both. Numerous books on the topic provide a "recipe" to help a person live to one hundred ten or to one hundred twenty or more years. The question that is often asked is whether such claims have any clinical credibility, and if so, what should you as a member of the interested public do if anything to extend your life expectancy and what are the implications?

First, it is important to understand certain basic concepts before the issue of life extension can be adequately discussed. The first is whether you are talking about increasing the average societal or population or individual life expectancy at the time of birth. The other is whether you are talking about increasing the expected life span of the whole human species. Held within these two concepts is whether any individual's life span can be extended, either at the time of birth to an unknown but on average longer period, or whether, if the potential life span of the whole human species can be extended, we can intervene in such a way that all humans in general or individuals within the species can live as close as possible to the maximum life span that can be achieved for the human species.

Once these factors are determined and a realistic assessment can be made as to what can be done in terms of how long we might live in the best circumstances, we can examine whether the potential options available are ethically sound or not—for the individuals involved or for society in general. The question is whether modern medicine and present knowledge allows us to promote a substantial shift in how long humans can live and, if so, what kinds of lives you might have if your life could be substantially extended.

As the child of an aged parent who is facing illnesses and the prospect of dying, the idea of life extension is usually focused on the specific issue of determining whether your loved one's individual life might be prolonged by effectively treating a specific illness or group of diseases. This is different from thinking about an endeavor to increase the potential life span of the human species. Or you might think about actions that might increase the general life span of the species and therefore indirectly improve that of your own loved one through some sort of life-enhancing formula.

Some might simplistically say that if you prevent your aged parent from dying of a heart attack by providing potentially life-saving cardiac (heart) surgery that is a form of life extension, because the time of death is being postponed in the individual whose life has been saved. Most would agree in the simple sense that is true, but that is not what is usually meant by life extension strategies. Those proponents usually mean that you must undertake major interventions in your lifestyle throughout your lifetime as the means of extending your life potential as an individual and propose that such changes on a general basis will increase the average life span of all or most members of society.

In many ways this has been happening at the societal level in many if not all parts of the world during the past century. The life expectancy at birth has increased substantially over the past few decades so that the numbers of elders living well into their eighties and nineties and occasionally exceeding one hundred years has become fairly common, especially in the developed world. But this is partially if not substantially due to a remarkable decline in the previously devastating loss of children before the age of immunization and the improvements in public health measures that provide our citizenry with reliable water supplies and ways of safely maintaining food products. The improvements in health care treatments such as antibiotics that have resulted in the decline in previously lethal infections that wiped out many members of a population as well as, for example, improvements in the treatment of cardiovascular disease have all had a beneficial effect on the number of years a person might be expected to live on average. There are still many individual variations due to a person's genetic makeup and good or not-so-good fortune.

Although health care professionals currently usually encourage improvements in lifestyle practices such as exercise, proper diet, and the elimination of external risk factors for disease such as cigarette smoking, these alone can only maximize your chances of reaching the biologically determined maximum that you have within you based on all your multiple genetic and biologic factors. The life extension movement suggests otherwise and has challenged some of the traditional principles and belief systems in health care and society to promote their goals. Of the potentially beneficial steps that individuals can take to enhance their chance of a long life, caloric restriction throughout one's lifetime seems to be one of the steps that have a degree of credibility. Those of us who have tried this throughout our lives realize that it is not the easiest thing to do especially in countries where the culture and the food industry promote eating in excess. Food and dining with family and friends are among the cornerstones of social interaction.

A while ago, I was invited to a conference called "Creating Very Old People: Individual Blessing or Societal Disaster?" I could not attend, but the topic made me reconsider the perpetual quest for longevity that has become an obsession in contemporary Western society. It is common these days to see organizations and clinics dedicated to "anti-aging" and to selling products for the same purpose. It has become a huge industry. We might question whether or not we should consider prolonging life at all costs. The June 2004 issue of the *Journals of Gerontology* was devoted to "Anti-Aging Medicine: The Hype and the Reality." It is worth considering the topic from the perspective of medical ethics and from the perspective of whether we would want this for our parents or for ourselves should the possibility realistically arise.

The grandfather of one of my colleagues died at the age of one hundred six, with only the last couple of years of life being totally dependent for care on others. He went to his hardware store, one of the first in Toronto, until the age of one hundred and sat around talking to customers.

My own father recently turned ninety-eight years old. Although he now needs some major help following a hip fracture a few years ago, he was until very recently able to enjoy a good movie, even the same one over and over, and a good meal, especially baked treats made by my wife. He can still enjoy people and have a good laugh.

I knew my father was still engaged in life when a year after he moved from New York, which was a few years ago, into a retirement home in Chicago, I asked him for *The New York Times* view on a current topic. It was my way of periodically (almost every week) checking his mental status in an indirect way.

He paused and said, "I don't get *The New York Times* anymore." I was shocked as my father, for most of his life, had read *The New York Times* every day. For many years during my adolescence he had a small side business delivering the *Times* in addition to reading it. From those years jumping off the back of the green Ford station wagon laden with hundreds of weighty Sunday *Times*, I not only got my feel of them and their content (as I folded the many sections into each other before delivery) but also learned to appreciate the special smell of the print they used. In fact, it took many minutes of washing with soap and water at the end of the morning's delivery to clean the highly staining ink from my hands. I asked my father why he didn't get the paper anymore, and his reply filled me with relief and optimism: "*The New York Times* has no local Chicago news, so I've changed to the *Tribune*." That was not bad for ninety years old.

When researchers and proponents of life extension talk about the subject, they are not referring to bypass surgery or dialysis at age eighty-five as a way of prolonging an individual's life as treatment of an illness. They are referring to proposals to substantially decrease the process and rate of aging. They are talking about not only increasing life expectancy, but also virtually eliminating or redefining the scourges of the aging process.

Life-extension proposals are not new; in fact, the idea of an elixir of life is almost as old as humanity itself. However, in a more contemporary approach, the classic 1981 book by Fries and Crapo, *Vitality and Aging*, suggests that a maximum biological human life span is just less than one hundred years, with some individuals living longer. A book by Pearson and Shaw in 1982, *Life Extension: A Practical and Scientific Approach*, and another one in 1984 by Walford, *Maximum Life Span*, argue that if people did the "right thing," they could increase the likelihood of meeting their biological maximum life span and also extend this age to perhaps one hundred twenty years or more, while remaining in relatively good health. It is interesting that a classical Jewish traditional blessing says, "You should live to one hundred twenty years." It comes from the Hebrew saying, attributed to the prophet Moses—and this existed long before the life-extension movement gained supporters or believers.

Walford's prescription for life extension as promoted in his book is a life-long, very low-calorie diet, which he parlayed into a second book called *Beyond the 120-Year Diet*. The irony is that Walford promotes severe calorie restriction when, in much of the world, insufficient caloric intake is one of the greatest public health problems. A comment at the time of Walford's first book from one of the reviewers from the *Harvard Medical School Letter* was, "He can't guarantee that his followers will live longer, but I would bet that it feels longer."

Recently there have been reports about another chemical agent or drug that seems to promote longevity, at least so far in mice, even older mice. As with other reports of this nature that make it into the literature and therefore make news from time to time, we must all await the real results, which may take years to sort out and then of course deal with the social implications of such advances should they prove to be verified.

One such study was reported in the July 2009 issue of the journal *Nature*. "When U.S. scientists treated old mice with rapamycin, it extended their expected life span by up to 38 percent. The findings ... raise the prospect of being able to slow down the aging process in older people. We believe this is the first convincing evidence that the aging process can be slowed and life span can be extended by a drug therapy starting at an advanced age," Professor Randy Strong of the University of Texas was quoted as saying.

However, a U.K. expert warned against using the drug to try to extend life span, as it can suppress immunity. Dr. Lynne Cox, a University of Oxford expert in aging, described the study as "exciting." She also said, "It is especially interesting that the drug was effective even when given to older mice, as it would be much better to treat aging in older people rather than using drugs long-term through life." However, she added, "In no way should anyone consider using this particular drug to try to extend their own life span, as rapamycin suppresses immunity."

In contrast to the proponents of life extension, Dr. Jay Olshansky, a prominent professor of public health at the University of Chicago, has been critical of such claims while acknowledging the excellent gains in life expectancy due to public health interventions and decreased incidence of serious life-shortening disease. According to Olshansky, much of what you read about prevention of aging is pure "snake oil" referring to the age-old practice of charlatans selling miraculous cures to the unknowing and gullible public. The original exponents of near-starvation diets, antioxidant therapy, and human growth hormone, he points out in his 2002 book, *The Quest for Immortality*, are all dead. But research into anything and everything that could stop aging is a booming industry. For the first time in human history, millions of people will grow old.

The real question is what if it were biologically possible to substantially increase the human life span, not just life expectancy at birth, so that vast numbers of people, by diet or drugs or some other combination of personal intervention, could live until one hundred twenty years old. What are the ethical implications of this possibility for individuals, families, the structure of society, and the planet?

Gulliver's Travels: Lessons to Be Learned?

When Jonathan Swift wrote *Gulliver's Travels*, he included the story of the Struldbruggs who were condemned to immortality accompanied not by perpetual health but by continuous decline. Of interest is Swift's concern about the effect of language on this immortal population. Because the language of their country was always in flux as is the case in most modern societies, the Struldbruggs of one age did not understand those of another; neither were they able, after two hundred years, to hold a real conversation (other than a few general salutations) with their neighbors—the non-life-extended mortals. Thus they lived like foreigners in their own country. Becoming disconnected from younger generations and their needs could lead to a serious conflict between generations.

The main ethical conflict in the life-extension paradigm to be considered by children or their parents is related to the ethical principle of distributive justice. How would a society decide who gets what if there were a substantial increase in a population that required a significant amount of resources? Very aged people, despite doing all the "right" things, will inevitably have the range of illnesses that now occur at an earlier age. The life-extension proposals do not suggest an elimination of disability and disease; they merely suggest a postponement of it. Will the younger generations be capable of providing the care to support this increasingly numerous and aged population? Will aged people, by necessity, form unique and defined social strata that are self-serving and self-sustaining?

One might ask the basic human and ethical question of whether or not it is the responsibility of each successive generation to take care of their elders. If so, what happens when a generation becomes too elderly themselves? Currently, parents take care of their aging parents while their children are busy with careers and having children of their own. What happens when mom can no longer take care of grandma, and daughter has to take care of both, as well as her new baby? Talk about a "sandwich" generation; this would be more like a multi-layered club sandwich generation.

Last, this question would have to be addressed: Can the planet sustain another generation or two of humans who, by nature, plunder the planet to survive? What degree of human narcissism would we be promoting if we undertook the process of life extension seriously? One of the realities that focus human energies is the idea of life limitation and death; to postpone this into a much further future might undermine man's creative motivations that are often governed by the knowledge of foreseeable and finite mortality.

Perhaps entitled Western scholars who are contemplating the possibilities of some sort of life-extension process would play a more useful role if they would focus on eliminating poverty and hunger and premature death, which affect much of humankind, rather than trying to squeeze a few more years from those who live in the richest countries.

In their book *Vitality and Aging*, Fries and Crapo describe their approach as "squaring the curve" rather than life extension. Instead of the percentage of the population declining steadily as age increases, they suggest that with improvements in lifestyle, sanitation, food, and public health, the curve can be squared with a much higher percentage of the population living to a certain age, rather than a much smaller percentage surviving beyond that point. In essence, individual quality of life is improved and lengthened, and time spent in a frail and declining state is shortened, without extending the overall life expectancy of a population—people live for just as long, they just live better lives. That is the state that most of us try to achieve, and those who care for aging parents seek interventions to achieve that goal for their parents and presumably for themselves sometime in the future when they themselves age.

Many scholars and clinical practitioners in the field of aging, like Olshansky, reject the concept of life extension, as it is a combination of "snake oil" and entrepreneurial greed. There are sound ethical reasons to reject it even if it were an attainable goal. As it is written in Ecclesiastes 3:1-8, "To everything there is a season ... a time to be born and a time to die"—and that time should not be postponed for another twenty, thirty, forty, or fifty mythical years.

Points to Remember

- We live in an age when life expectancy at birth has been greatly extended compared to the time our parents were our age.
- With the increase in life expectancy, it is easy to forget that, even with modern medical technology, each life has its upper limit.
- Each of us will probably struggle with our own mortality and the possible choices between maximizing our life's length or its quality—at times the two may not be congruent with each other.
- When it comes to our parents, we will often have to decide whether any extension in the length of life is worth what has to be done to achieve the extra hours, weeks, or months and sometimes years—weighing quantity as opposed to quality.
- One of the great ethical challenges that children of aging parents will often contend with is when to say enough is enough, even in the face of medical technologies that might offer some fragment of hope for more time, but not necessarily the kind of time our beloved parent may desire or is able to express to us.

The Timeline of Decline

It might be much easier to come to terms with the reality of the future if you could anticipate the timeline of decline of your older loved one. I have often heard children of aging parents ask, "What can I expect so I can plan for it?" which is a common notion in a world in which we love to plan for the future.

Although there might be a common trajectory that many people go through in their later years with incrementally declining function, it is not uncommon for individuals to leap from one stage or level of function to another suddenly for reasons that cannot always be predicted. For example, a person with mild dementia who is functioning adequately at home with a modicum of help a few hours a day could, after a serious illness that affects her cognitive (mental) function, require full-time live-in help or a permanent nursing home admission.

To give a sense of what a conceptualized timeline of incremental decline might look like, I will provide the example of my father whose timeline has been very different from that of my late mother. In her case, she went from fully functioning and independent to completely dependent, hospitalized, and then a short palliative period until she succumbed to her illness in a relatively short time. Her story when contrasted with my father's are examples of the spectrum that family members might experience as they try to make the best of their loved one's aging and declining process so that they can take steps to do the best and right things when the challenges occur.

My father was fully independent and functioning into his late eighties when my mother over a short period developed first a mini-stroke followed by a major stroke, which resulted in total paralysis of one side of her body, and then a terrible cascade of events that led to her death. The family decision to decline further medical intervention including tube feeding was one of the greatest emotionally challenging struggles my father and sister and I had to make. We had never as a family faced such a decision before, even though I had done so many times in my professional career.

For the first few years after his wife's death, my father seemed to manage in the small bungalow he had shared with her and the rest of the family for many decades. He was alone, yet he had a few kind neighbors and one devoted sister who lived in the city but not close by. He did not want to continue attending the senior center that he had attended with my mother as he said it "caused him to cry whenever he entered it and recalled the times they had together there." We tried to encourage him but realized that his general desire to be alone would be the way he was going to live. He seemed to be cognitively intact and was still doing his own banking, shopping and directing a stock portfolio, and driving competently.

When my sister or I visited, although the house was messy, we observed that it was not more so than it would have been had my mother not struggled all of her life to bring some order to it. My sister shared the credit card account with my father, so she could track his supermarket shopping charges. They seemed to have a steady rhythm of purchases. When we visited, there was always a reasonable quantity and variety of food in the refrigerator. He had a few long-standing neighbors who would kindly supply us with updates on his well-being, so things seemed to be going reasonably well for a few years.

Then we started getting the phone calls: "I just got another parking ticket for being on the wrong side of the street." The first time it seemed to be an anomaly, part of the alternate side of the street parking problem in his neighborhood that was meant to allow for street cleaning and to which he adhered carefully. Then it happened again.

On my next trip, I spoke to a neighbor who admitted to me that he would see my father sometimes move the car to the correct side of the street and then a few hours later move it back to where it had been, which was going to be the wrong side of the street. Sometimes he would try gently to correct my father, but it did not always succeed. During that visit the house seemed to be in greater disarray, and some of the food in the refrigerator was moldy, and there was a decreased variety of foods.

My sister Diti and I talked to each other and then to him. I had tried a few years earlier when things were going reasonably well to move him to Toronto and went through the immigration details, which eventually were approved. After a visit to start arranging the move, he called and said he changed his mind because "taxes were too high in Canada," and he was worried he would not be able to drive.

No amount of counter-information could change his mind. Now Diti and I were confronted with what to do if he could not manage. We spoke to him on a visit, and he refused to think about moving to Chicago where Diti lives. In our usual respectful way, after discussing the reasons, we deferred to him. He as usual refused any help in the house for cleaning—he was still going down into the basement using the trap door in a closet and negotiating the narrow stairs to use the washing machine and dryer. We found lots of his clothes hanging on a wooden dryer as he said the machine did not do such a good job, and he didn't want to have it repaired.

Then the visit occurred that changed the pathway. We were visiting for his birthday and went to a restaurant to celebrate with his sister. At the end of an enjoyable meal, while his sister and brother-in-law went to the restrooms, he looked at Diti and me and said, "How did I get here?"

When we got to the house, we found it a disaster with food crumbs and partially eaten bread and crackers everywhere and mouse droppings along the floor in the dining area. His bed looked like it had not been made in weeks and there were bottles of vodka nearby and a whole range of over-the-counter pain relievers as well as some sleeping medications. He told us he needed them because of his back pain.

We sat him down and said to him, not in an asking voice, "Daddy, things are dangerous here, we are worried about you, and we want to move you to Chicago." We expected a strong negative reply, but instead he looked down and said, "Okay, I am willing to try it. But do not sell the house."

Diti found a nice retirement home near where she lived, and within a few weeks she drove him and the most critical papers and belongings to Chicago where he moved into a retirement home. With a proper geriatric medical assessment, his pain issues were addressed, all the over-the-counter sleeping aids and inappropriate medications were discontinued, and his apparent mental impairment was addressed through the prescription of Aricept, a drug that had been on the market for only a few years.

With all these steps including a most supportive living environment with proper meals and social activities, which he started attending, and my sister's frequent visits, he blossomed. I visited and could not believe the transformation.

Then after not quite two months he told my sister he wanted to go back home because he felt so much better. She convinced him knowing his psychology that having paid for the retirement home for three months that he would not forgo the payment and stay until the time was up. In the meanwhile he was not driving even though he periodically asked to do so, as the car was in Diti's driveway. When he brought the subject up, Diti would explain problems with insurance but would take him for a drive to some rural area and let him drive. After a few minutes he usually said it was enough, and she took over again. Gradually the requests to drive diminished and then finally stopped.

One night he called Diti over because he was having a terrible bout of constipation, a recurrent theme in his life. She stayed with him throughout the night administering laxatives and yogurt. Finally in the morning he had his bowel movement, declared that she had "saved his life," and told her to "sell the house in Brooklyn." The process of emptying the house of its contents was a challenge for the two of us. But we found many wonderful items of memorabilia including letters and pictures that brought back our childhood to us and gave us some insights into both our mother and father and allowed us to close the house after it was sold.

My father was now permanently living in Chicago in a retirement home—the next in the common stages of decline in which difficult decisions by family members have to be made.

Since that move, his life in Chicago has been beset by a number of typical events often faced by families of older people who have decision-making challenges with ethical underpinnings. We decided to have a discussion with my father about his future wishes for care should something terrible happen to him. I had such a discussion with him sometime after my mother had died, and he had clearly indicated that he would not want the kind of *heroics* that she had experienced during the last period of her illness and would not want to suffer. We had the discussion again, this time with my sister present, and he reiterated the same principles. That helped us understand the values that he ascribed to and which we would have to call on in decision-making during illnesses he had later.

During the past few years, we struggled with major clinical and ethical decision-making. One event was his sudden need for heart bypass surgery after we had believed it was not something he would consider based on previous discussions. But under the circumstances in which the events leading to the decision occurred and the fact that he was mentally sufficiently competent despite his mild cognitive impairment to make the decision—he went through the procedure with flying colors.

Then the issue became his inability to take his medications properly, which resulted in getting some help at the retirement home to give him his medications according to schedule, but he was otherwise able to live alone in his suite and participate in the activities he enjoyed in the building. Diti visited frequently, and I called usually once a week when I would do a Mini-Mental State–type exam by asking him what was "in the news"—as he read a newspaper every day.

Then the fall in the middle of the night, the fractured hip, the stormy postoperative course, the state of confusion during the attempted rehabilitation program, and then the decision to return to his own suite rather than moving him to the assisted living level of the retirement home, but now with full-time live-in help. A new decision had to be made, and we made it based on what we believed he would want and with his input to the best of his ability, which eventually after he had recovered from the trauma of the surgical period, concurred with our plan. He was now living with full-time help but with that arrangement managing to stay in his own suite. His needs for personal care grew but were attended to.

The next challenge and a common theme that children of aging parents have to face is an acute respiratory infection (pneumonia). For my father, this resulted in hospitalization and a period in which first his survival and then his ability to eat came into question. At one point his physician, who had diagnosed what he thought was aspiration pneumonia, raised the specter of a feeding tube without discussing the issue with us—working under the assumption physicians commonly hold that if they thought it was *dangerous* to eat by mouth, there was no alternative to a permanent feeding tube.

When we discovered that this was the physician's way of thinking, we informed him that our father had clearly indicated when he was cognitively in full control of his faculties that he would not accept a feeding tube and would either succumb to his illness or take the chances of eating by mouth even if it were a modified diet.

Despite the physician's differing opinion and focus on risk, we gradually introduced yogurt and then more types of food to my father. He was discharged back to the retirement home in our care, and one of the wonderful pictures I have of him is eating honey cake that my wife, Gilda, had baked for him, which he loved and was able to eat without turning a hair. The next time he acquired a flulike respiratory infection, despite a cough that sounded frightening, we decided to keep him in his suite and treat him supportively, and that too he survived without the rigors and risks of hospitalization.

He is now at the age of ninety-eight, living with full-time help in the same retirement home, dependent in many domains of everyday living but still able to recognize those that matter to him, enjoy food, and take part on occasion in a community lunch program and social programs run by the facility. He is not independently mobile. Diti and I know that *something* will occur one day that may be the *final* illness, but we have a reasonable idea what matters to him most. Although we know the emotional effects will not diminish just because he is ninety-eight, we are as prepared as any children can be for the future.

Our father's story is an example of the experience that many children of aging parents confront. In some ways the gradual decline is a blessing in that it, in contrast to the sudden catastrophic illness and death of our mother, allows for children to have a longer period of life and shared experiences with a loved one. But the long-term challenges and strain on caregiving children and their families can be substantial and must be addressed in order for the final outcomes to be as good as you might hope for.

Common, Everyday Activities: Driving

"My father is angry with you and with me for bringing him to you." We were just starting a follow-up appointment after a previous geriatric assessment and a number of investigations for my patient Ben's problem with cognitive decline. The medical resident had just finished the evaluation in my ambulatory geriatric teaching clinic, and together we were interviewing the patient, who was accompanied by his caring and devoted daughter.

"Generally his condition is stable," the resident said in our preliminary discussion after he did his evaluation and before entering the room with the patient, "with no real decline in his mental or physical function; and if anything his Mini-Mental State Examination has gone up a bit, but nothing significant."

I entered the examining room with the resident after she reported her findings. I reviewed the medications and ascertained from Ben what he was taking, which his daughter confirmed. Then Ben started with an angry edge to his voice, "I must get my license back. There is no reason that I can't drive. I am losing money because I can't visit my buildings to check that everything is okay and speak to the superintendents. How do I know if they are doing their job?" The daughter's expression said it all—he was fixated on the subject of his driving.

I asked him where the properties were. "In north Toronto and out east a bit. I have only a few low rises left. I need to see them to know they are okay. I can't do this without my car." I asked him if there was another way for him to get to the places he needed without a car.

He looked at me quizzically.

I reminded him, "Ben, last time you were here, I explained why I had to report you to the Ministry of Transportation. We discussed the cost of running your car compared to the cost of taking taxis to wherever you need to go, especially when you said that you do not use the car a lot."

His daughter looked at him and said, "Dad, we talked about this as well last week, and I showed you the cost of insurance and upkeep and gas; and we figured you could take hundreds of taxis a year for those costs."

Ben looked at her and then at me and said, "You don't understand. In my business I have to visit the buildings to make sure everything is okay and not having a car makes it impossible. I don't understand why you took my license away. I have been driving for more than sixty years."

The patient was angry with his children for some months and expressed his anger at me each time he came. But over time as the taxi system was put into place and he found he could travel when he wanted to, which became in fact less and less often as his needs decreased, the driving issue waned as one that caused enormous strife between the patient and his family.

This scenario in one form or another is played out a few times a month if not more often in my once-a-week half-day geriatric assessment clinic. The issue of driving is one of the most difficult and contentious challenges that physicians have to face, especially those of us who deal with the increasingly elderly population. Sometimes the problem stems from the fact that the person may believe he or she is going to the physician for one reason, even if it is memory problems, never contemplating that driving may be curtailed at the end of the interview. This can be a disturbing and shocking experience, even if you as the family member are convinced and maybe happy that finally a doctor has acted on what you have been concerned about for many months or longer. On occasion, I am asked to provide a second opinion because the patient believes the original doctor for some reason erred or was age-biased and that coming to me would reverse the decision—this reversal has happened rarely over many years of such experiences.

The ethical issues involved are usually understood by the family members and sometimes by the patients in question, even when they deny that the ethical principle applies to them. Potential harm to themselves and others overrides personal benefit and convenience. The physician's duty may seem in conflict with that of the patient and that of the public. However, like in other public health issues, such as the mandatory reporting of certain contagious diseases, society has established the priorities to the public rather than the individual in such situations. Safe driving is no different.

If you were to look back over the course of the decline of your parent's life, it often starts with issues that are not dramatic but portend the future dependency and loss of function that often occurs with aging. In contrast to profound and at times almost existential questions such as maximizing life or extending it, relatively simple losses of ability may be indicators of what the future holds in store. What might appear to be in a different category from the deep questions of life and death can have a profound effect on older individuals and you and other members of your family.

Some issues can be pivotal events in the process of aging and loss of one's self-esteem and independence. A commonly experienced event such as the loss of the driver's license is an example of how an apparently simple activity can have profound meaning and effect on an older person's world as well as on your relationship to your parent. It can affect your need to affirm that you have been protective of your loved one and have acted ethically to the community in which you are also a member.

Problems with driving are a common phenomenon and an increasing challenge to families and physicians as the number of the elderly has grown in the population. One report in 2008 suggests that many people with early Alzheimer's disease or mild dementia may initially be able to drive safely. As reported in a Reuters article by Joene Hendry: "Their driving skills predictably decline over one to two years to a level that often precludes safe driving," according to Dr. Brian R. Ott of the Alzheimer's Disease and Memory Disorders Center at Rhode Island Hospital in Providence. "Red flags that indicate it's time to take away the keys include driving too slowly, being confused or undecided at intersections, getting lost in familiar locations, failing to observe traffic signs and signals, and being in an at-fault motor vehicle accident," Ott told Reuters.

According to a report from the Massachusetts Institute of Technology's AgeLab, drivers with dementia are staying on the road too long. According to a study from MIT AgeLab, Boston University, and The Hartford Financial Services Group, people with Alzheimer's disease continued to drive for an average of ten months longer than their caregivers felt was safe. Depending on the jurisdiction, the requirements to report the person to the driving ministry or regulatory body may vary.

The rules from the Ministry of Transportation in Ontario, for example, are not as clear about cognitive impairment as a cause for reporting to them compared to other neurological disorders, such as epilepsy. The wording that addresses the reporting issue says, "Every legally qualified medical practitioner shall report to the Registrar of Motor Vehicles ... who, in the opinion of the medical practitioner, has a condition that *may* make it dangerous for the person to operate a motor vehicle."

The challenge for physicians is that our reporting duty is mandatory and the use of the term *may*. Therefore, most physicians, who are aware of the increased likelihood of accidents involving people with cognitive impairment or dementia, even if the person seems to be managing reasonably well and has been accident free, feel that they must report the person to the Ministry offices. This approach puts the onus on the Ministry to decide whether to remove the driver's license. Therefore, it is not the doctor who takes away the license, but it is the doctor who must report the concerns and the clinical findings—it would be rare for a license to be maintained if the physician fills out the form with a diagnosis of dementia. In California, the state requires physicians to submit a confidential report to the county health department when an individual is diagnosed as having a dementing illness. This information is forwarded to the Department of Motor Vehicles that is authorized to take action against the driving privileges of any individual who is unable to safely operate a motor vehicle.

One option that sometimes allows for a deferral of the decision in borderline situations is to refer the person to one of the third-party driving assessment programs such as DriveAble, which exists across Canada. Similar programs exist in other jurisdictions in North America. A good resource for the United States can be found on the National Highway Traffic Safety Administration website's older drivers program section: http://www.nhtsa.dot.gov/portal/site/nhtsa/menuitem.31176b9b03647a189ca8e410dba046a0/

Organizations and programs such as DriveAble do a reliable in-depth assessment of the driving abilities of the person in question. Their final reports may inform the decision about notification to the Ministry of Transportation and/or their final decision. (The cost currently is $495 in Canada. Sometimes individuals resent having to pay to keep their license and do not understand that the program is separate from the government and therefore not biased and is funded by the fees it charges.)

I often recommend that third-party route, and if the outcome is successful, everyone seems to feel that it was an investment worth making. In some U.S. jurisdictions, the Department of Motor Vehicles does this kind of test before deciding on whether or not to remove the driving license.

Losing driving privileges is a serious blow to a person's mobility, independence, and sense of dignity. However, driving is not a right but a privilege, and physicians are obligated to serve the public safety by their role, however uncomfortable and contentious that might be. The important issue is dealing with the underlying anger associated with the loss of a driver's license in an older person. For you and your family it may indicate what may be the beginning of an inexorable decline in potential independence and function for your aging parent. The timeline is unpredictable, but the alert flags have been raised.

Points to Remember

- Many older people feel that driving is their right, but if they have dementia, they do not have the insight to recognize their impairments on the road.
- Losing one's driver's license can be emotionally devastating and can lead to problems with mobility of the older person and decrease the sense of and state of independence.
- It can be especially difficult for loving family members to report the driving problems to the doctor when they know the likelihood of their elderly loved one's losing the ability to drive.
- A logical review of the financial benefits of giving up one's driver's license and car and using taxis instead may have some effect on the person depending on his or her degree of cognition but is often unconvincing in removing the anger at having the driver's license removed.
- Occasionally a government-run or third-party driving assessment may conclude that the person is still safe to drive. If so, the person may continue to drive as long as the assessment is repeated on a periodic basis, such as yearly.

Romance and Sex

The daughter and her father, the patient referred to me, were sitting in my office. He had been living in a retirement home without the need for assisted living for well over a year. The main medical problem revolved around some mild memory impairment and a suggestion of a negative or depressed mood. The clinical evaluation did not suggest a significant degree of cognitive impairment or mood disorder that would require medication. During the interview, the daughter mentioned that her father had a "girlfriend" at the home and that there were some issues with her.

Her father piped in, "And they won't even invite her to their house when they have me over. It isn't nice, you know. Her family is considerate of me, and my family acts as if she doesn't exist."

The daughter appeared uncomfortable as her father continued, "You'd think that they could at least accept her even if they don't like her very much. It is my choice, isn't it?"

We decided that the clinic visit was not a good milieu to continue the discussion, but I offered the daughter and her siblings (she had two in the city) assistance if they wanted to discuss the issue with a social worker or anyone else.

Romance and sex are powerful human forces—some of the most powerful that exist. There has been a lot of mythology around the natural loss of interest and ability for romance and sex as one ages—the truth being that this is not necessarily the case in many older individuals, including those in their very late years. The challenge is: what do you and your family do if and when your older parent enters into a late-life romantic or sexual relationship that you are not emotionally or intellectually prepared for?

The question might be, "Who decides when elderly individuals wherever they may be living should or can participate in romantic or sexual relationships?" If they are mentally competent the question is easy to answer—they decide, whether you and your family necessarily are happy with the decision. If there is some question about mental or emotional abilities or competency the question may not be as easy to answer. So many issues come to play, including personalities, the individual needs of people for romance and sexuality, opportunities, the views and values of those around us, including you and your family. With all of these issues there are underlying ethical considerations that cannot be overlooked.

A while ago, I was visiting an Ontario nursing home that had requested help developing its ethics program. The unit nurse said they had a difficult case based on a sexual issue and that they were unsure of what to do. "We have already had a few cases like this, and we expect that we'll have more cases, and we want some kind of standardized, or at least consistent and agreed-to, approach."

This was clearly a hot topic, and everyone had an opinion. The case involved two individuals living in the nursing home. They resided on the same floor. Peter, age eighty-six, has mild dementia, diabetes, and heart disease, with a previous stroke. He has been in the home just over a year. He doesn't require assistance for most of his activities of daily living and is charming, sociable, and caring. Peter became lonely after his wife died, which was about seven years before he was admitted to the nursing home. He had a relationship with another woman, starting about two years after his wife died, which lasted for a couple of years, but for the past three years he has been alone, which contributed to the decision to arrange admission for him at the home.

Loretta's situation is a bit more complicated. She has moderate dementia and has been at the home for a year longer than Peter. She can still do her own dressing, toileting, and grooming but needs guidance in what clothes to wear. But once provided, she can put them on herself correctly. She is forgetful of dates and people until she meets them a few times. However, she recognizes her family, the staff, many of the residents, and, of course, Peter.

At one of the afternoon socials with refreshments, music, and dancing, Peter approached Loretta. By the end of the afternoon, it was clear there was some chemistry between them. One of the social workers commented, "It is pretty common for residents at the get-togethers to share various social activities, and dancing is one of the ways people connect in a warm and convivial way. However, it usually does not carry over as it has with Loretta and Peter."

One of the nurses at the meeting continued, "It is interesting to see the response. Peter's son and daughter think this is wonderful for both Peter and Loretta and have not seen their father so happy in a long time. Loretta's two daughters are mortified at the thought of their elderly mother, who has been widowed for more than ten years, having relations with someone they perceive as a stranger. They feel that, because she has a diagnosis of probable Alzheimer's dementia, she cannot possibly make decisions of this kind, and therefore Peter is taking advantage of her. The family has threatened legal action if the home does not do something to prevent this from occurring."

I asked about the staff's response, and the nursing administrator and the unit's social worker summarized, "The staff is of two minds. Some think this is great and have watched the relationship grow in a way that seems absolutely genuine; they recognize both Peter and Loretta are flourishing in their new relationship and think everyone, including the children, should be supporting it." Other staff members think it is not right that Peter and Loretta be allowed to continue the relationship. Their main concern is that Loretta has dementia and that she is unable to make such an important decision about romantic or sexual relations with someone. Given her perceived inability, they believe that she should not be allowed to partake in such deeply personal activities.

I explained to the staff the importance of trying to address this situation in an ethical framework in addition to any other considerations to make sure we all understand the issues and how the involved parties might interpret them.

The first issue that must be considered is: who is, and who should be, making the decision about a romantic and potentially sexual relationship? We had to make sure that we agreed collectively that the autonomy of the people we care for in the geriatric and long-term care system should be an important, if not the only, focal point of decision-making. Out of that assumption we had to agree that unless proven otherwise, Peter and Loretta have the ability to decide with whom they want to have a relationship. Only if one or both of them could not act in any reasonably autonomous fashion would we have to remove from them the ability to make their own decisions and direct those to their lawful surrogates, who in this case would be their children.

The other issue related to this is the question of what kinds of decisions are being made. The usual way the principles of ethics are used is within the domain of health care decisions or those concerning assets and resources. It is not clear if personal relationships can easily be interpreted under the ethical principles framework.

At this point, the nurses raised the issue of capacity in decision-making by asking, "How can a person with Alzheimer's disease be allowed to make such a decision?" Years ago we used to assume that if a person had a diagnosis of Alzheimer's disease, he or she was incapable of making any of his or her own decisions. The idea of global incapacity as the manifestation of dementias of any kind has long been dispelled. In general, the concept of domains of competence, or incompetence, is the current approach to capacity in decision-making. As an example that everyone should be able to understand, the financial cognitive capacity to supervise an investment portfolio is different from the ability to choose one's clothes for the day.

We shouldn't be surprised at the response of Loretta's children. They surely want only the best for their mother, and their reaction is understandable. But they need to better understand their role as surrogate decision makers. They are in this role to make only those decisions their mother is incapable of making. As long as the decisions made by Loretta to have romantic or sexual interactions with Peter do not seem wildly out of character, they have no ethical grounds or, as it stands, legal grounds to question Loretta's capacity unless her behavior is inappropriate given the circumstances.

The law would normally be translated to support the ethical principle; therefore, usually people are legally allowed to make such important personal decisions unless it is clear that they are incapable of doing so or there is a significant risk to their well-being by being allowed to do so. This does not appear to be the case in the present situation.

Can Sex and Romance Be Prohibited in a Long-Term Care Facility or Nursing Home?

The second issue is this: Is it inappropriate for clients of a geriatric facility who are experiencing dementia to have romantic or sexual interactions? Romantic and sexual feelings are long learned and deeply entrenched, along with individual inhibitions and personality. There is nothing to suggest romantic or sexual desires or inclinations are any less valid when experienced by a person with dementia than when experienced by a person who is cognitively intact. It can be argued that a desire for intimate relations is no different than a desire for certain types of food or a good laugh. To deprive a person of being able to manifest his or her romantic and sexual interests in a mutually acceptable and congruent fashion is unreasonable ethically and does not have any obvious merit legally.

Both Loretta's children and the staff need to understand that, despite her cognitive impairment, Loretta seems to be able to find the important and satisfying associations of affection and physicality. The staff and her daughters agree she appears to be happy with the relationship. If everyone can understand that, for Loretta, this relationship is a positive experience and not something she needs to be protected from, perhaps some headway can be made with the reluctant daughters.

After much discussion, the staff agreed there was an ethical imperative and humane obligation to promote goodwill among the family members and staff in this romantic tale. The social worker and nurse agreed open and supportive discussions with the two daughters would be worthwhile.

The last major challenge for the staff and administration is how to provide the couple with the privacy to pursue their romantic relationship if there seemed to be a need for that step. The administrator agreed to look into developing a room that would be inviting to couples that seek a place to express their affections privately. Because Peter and Loretta are both acting in a way that is rational, and typical, their families and the care home staff are obliged to do everything possible to allow Peter and Loretta the freedom to enjoy their lives as they choose, and to the fullest.

If it weren't for the fact that romance and sexuality were not among the most important aspects of human endeavor, we would not spend much of our developmental and adult years seeking out and enjoying activities related to our sexual and romantic attributes. It is naïve to assume that older people including those with problems with cognition would forget about or not need those same satisfactions, either in thought or action that consumed so much of their lives. Some societies are more open than others in accepting and addressing issues related to sexuality in older persons. In North America we continue to share a bit of prudishness about human sexuality, especially as it affects older people.

In the first clinical scenario, while I was having the discussion with the daughter about her opinion about her father's "friend," I asked her if her boyfriends were always liked by her parents when she was growing up and if the boyfriends and girlfriends of her young adult children were always pleasing to her when they were adolescents and now as adults as neither of them were married. She agreed that at times there were concerns, but as a parent she had long ago decided along with her husband that they would state their case if appropriate (if asked for example) and then let their children follow through with their own decisions. They realized that their children might not achieve what they wanted if the parents took strong positions.

Being an adult child of older parents who are manifesting their personalities in a romantic and sexual way may not be easy. Many factors come into play including fear of their being disappointed or hurt, complications that may occur in any complex personal relationship, and concerns about money and other financial implications that may occur depending on the outcome of the relationship. The goal of fulfilling the beneficent role of a caring child often requires that you project yourself into the mind and feelings of the person you love and try to understand how important a romantic and sexual relationship might be. Then the challenge is to find ways to provide care and love while supporting the heart and soul of your parent.

New Views on the Subject of Late-Life Romance and Sex

A great deal has been written recently, and there have been some outstanding media representations about the issue of romance and sex in the later years and its effect on individuals with dementia and their loved ones. This subject might resonate in your own family situation, so it is worth noting some major changes in approach and attitude to the topic.

As noted in an article in the May 13, 2008, issue of Canada's *Medical Post* entitled, "Is It Ever Too Late for Love and Romance?" the recognition of the issue is supported by Sarah Polley's recent film *Away from Her* starring Gordon Pinsent and Julie Christie. The film is an example of dealing with a complex and difficult subject in a way that led to the film being a box office success and an Oscar contender.

It was in the context of my own clinical experiences with late-life romance and the conflict that often occurs among family members that I noted with great interest and satisfaction an article in the November 18, 2007, *New York Times* by Kate Zernike entitled "Love in the Time of Dementia." She noted, "Former Justice Sandra Day O'Connor's husband, suffering from

Alzheimer's disease, has a romance with another woman, and the former justice is thrilled—even visits with the new couple while they hold hands on the porch swing—because it is a relief to see her husband of fifty-five years so content."

With the exponential growth of the older population, we will have to develop new approaches and attitudes about what is being called by some *old love*, in contrast to *young love* about which so much has been written for eons. As noted in the *Times* article, "This is right up there in terms of the cutting-edge ethical and cultural issues of late-life love," said Dr. Thomas R. Cole, Director of the McGovern Center for Health, Humanities and the Human Spirit at the University of Texas and author of a cultural history of aging. "We need moral exemplars, not to slavishly imitate, but to help us identify ways of being in love when you're older."

Cole reminds readers, "It [love and romance] once conjured images that were distasteful or even scary: the dirty old man, the erotic old witch." But he goes on, "As life expectancy increases, and a generation more sexually liberated begins to age, nursing homes are being forced to confront an increase in sexual activity." Despite the stereotypes, researchers who study emotions across the life span say old love is in many ways more satisfying than young love—even as it is also more complex, as the O'Connor example shows.

"There's a difference between love as it is presented in movies and music as this jazzy sexy thing that involves bikini underwear and what love actually turns out to be," said the psychologist Mary Pipher, whose book *Another Country* looks at the emotional life of elderly people. "The really interesting script isn't that people like to have sex. The really interesting script is what people are willing to put up with," she writes. "Young love is about wanting to be happy," she said. "Old love is about wanting someone else to be happy."

Not everyone would show the emotionally generous response that Justice O'Connor did. As Dr. Cole said, "I have many examples in my mind of people who are just as jealous, just as infantile, just as filled with irrationality when they fall in love in their seventies and eighties as she is self-transcendent."

Do films like *Away from Her* anticipate a greater awareness, understanding, and acceptance of late-life romance including romance for those with dementia and other cognitively altering illnesses? The challenge for each of us who is the loving child of aging parents and for the long-term care industry and for society is to incorporate the realities of the range of lives and actions that elders have within them and find ways to deal with them in the most humane, supportive, and loving way possible.

Points to Remember

- Late-life romance in aging parents is something that children may have to contend with. It may be a challenge to find ways to turn the experience into something positive and meaningful and with which children can accept. It means overcoming deep-seated biases, fears, and stereotypes.
- Health care professionals and children of aged people have made enormous strides in understanding how to approach late-life romance and sex.
- Despite the changes, there are still many barriers to overcome that will allow late-life romance and sexual expression in those with cognitive impairment to be accepted as a normal part of the long-term care/nursing home setting.

4

Decision-Making: The Individual and the Surrogate Decision Maker

Angela sat at the end of the table with her father, Lorenzo, and sister Lisa on each side of her. Members of the health care team sat opposite, not by design to suggest alternate sides of the discussion, but it appeared to reflect the conflict that seemed to be developing.

"My mother, Maria, has been here for six months, and you are not only starving her to death, but you have failed to monitor her brain tumor as you should."

The staff was expecting an attack, so they were not surprised by the strong nature of the remarks.

They listened as she continued, "They told me at the general hospital when she was transferred to your palliative care unit that she would die in a few months at the most, and her care should be supportive. I knew that we had to agree to those terms, but I am not happy with the result of that decision. I am speaking on behalf of my father and sister when I ask you to please increase the dose of her steroids, send her for another CT scan, and arrange for another consultation with the neurosurgeon who operated on her. I want to know what other treatment can be provided for her to make her better."

The staff included the facility's ethicist because administrators had called on him to assist in dealing in a constructive fashion with the family. They had been struggling for many weeks with clear dissatisfaction expressed by Angela, although when the patient's husband and the other daughter, Lisa, were visiting without Angela in attendance, they seemed to be appreciative of the care Maria was receiving. Every now and then, Lisa would mention to a nurse that Angela was sometimes excessively critical and forceful, but she and her father appreciated her efforts to get the best care for Maria. Lorenzo once, while sitting alone by Maria's bed with tears in his eyes, spoke quietly to the nurse and asked why his wife could not just die peacefully rather than having her death drawn out with no ability to acknowledge or communicate with the family. He said, "We have been married for fifty-eight years, and I do not think she would want to be kept like this, she was so full of life and humor."

At the meeting, the attending physician explained, as she had in the past, that the effect of increased steroids on the tumor was unlikely to substantially improve the mother's condition and the likelihood of her waking up again as Angela had hoped for was not likely especially because the amount of steroids that Angela was talking about had failed to have any beneficial effect some months previously. At that time the staff in concert with the family had decided to taper somewhat the steroid dose to avoid the serious potential side effects, which included severe bleeding from the stomach, and which had been a problem some years before because of an ulcer. The doctors were concerned that the ulcer could be reactivated despite medications to try to prevent this from happening.

As for improving Maria's appetite, it was already a few months since Maria was able to take anything by mouth, and the feeding tube, which had been put in temporarily, was still a point of contention for Angela and her family—they didn't agree on it but as per their family pattern, Angela's determined views governed the decision-making.

The neurosurgeon had been called about the request for a repeat consultation but felt that it was of no value. He had done the surgery and found the large malignant tumor inoperable and had referred Maria for palliative radiation therapy, which resulted in a few months of benefit before the tumor started growing again. The surgeon felt that with the symptoms that she had (being virtually in a coma for many weeks), there would be no benefit from a repeated CT scan or repeat consultation. He had agreed to meet with the family if it was felt that his opinion might help the family deal with the reality of the situation.

Angela said, "I do not want my mother to see that neurosurgeon as he already has his pre-formed opinion. I want to see someone else who could look at my mother with fresh eyes."

In the meeting the ethicist asked Angela why she was pushing so hard for all these tests.

"I want to do the best for my mother. I think that she should have all the treatments that can be provided, even if it only means a few days or weeks more life for her and even if she doesn't wake up. While there is life, there is hope, you know, and I want to make sure she lives for as long as possible," Angela told the group.

The ethicist turned to Lorenzo and asked, "You have been married to Maria for almost sixty years. I would assume that you know your wife pretty well. Even if you may not have spoken about her deep-seated wishes about life and death, do you think she would want to be kept alive like this?" It was clear that there was a strong family dynamic going with Angela staring at her father in a way that showed she was hoping he would reflect her position.

"I am not sure what Maria would have wanted because we never talked about this, of course. But when her first cousin was sick in coma from a terrible stroke, Maria often asked why everyone was trying so hard to keep her alive. She believed strongly in God and the afterlife, so dying was not such a terrible thing for her. But that was about someone else, so I can't say what she would have wanted." While Lorenzo was speaking, Lisa unconsciously was nodding in agreement.

The ethicist wondered if the position taken by Angela was one that Lorenzo and Lisa were willing to accept, even if they did not completely agree with her or whether they believed that perhaps what she wanted was reasonable under the circumstances. As it turned out in this case, the conflict resolved itself when over a period of two days, Maria's condition deteriorated, the level of consciousness declined rapidly, and she died without any dramatic interventions being undertaken when it became clear to all including Angela that all options other than comfort measures were unrealistic. At this point her father clearly indicated that he wanted the death to be as gentle as possible.

For you to be prepared for many of the challenges that will be faced when assisting your older loved ones, you and your family need to understand some of the ethical and legal principles that determine the process of substitute decision-making. It is not as simple as many seem to believe. If anything it can be among the most daunting of tasks—making critical decisions on behalf of someone who is dearly loved and for whom important and at times life-determining decisions have to be made.

Throughout the life of all individuals, decisions are made. Some are minor and deal with the everyday and often mundane events that we all experience. In addition, we have more important decisions that all of us must face that can have a monumental effect on the essence of our lives, on our families, and on what will happen to us and to those we love. Among the relatively normal decisions include where we choose to live and study and the nature of the education or work we pursue. Also included is the choice of a marriage partner or the choice to not go the traditional route of marriage and family structure but some other option that is becoming easier and more widespread in most Western jurisdictions. For those who choose family relationships of whatever nature, the challenges embodied in such relationships are often myriad and complex and may include the nature and type of relationship, communication styles, whether the relationship will endure external or internal challenges or not, and if the latter what will happen to previously formed relationships as members of the family reconfigure themselves emotionally and structurally.

If children are involved, parents struggle with the decisions as they relate to offspring: education, partners, at what stage parental guidance is no longer wished for or needed, and all the various combinations and permutations of parent-child dynamics.

With the aging of a parent, what had in the past been a traditional dynamic of decision-making may alter first in terms of the relevant power or primacy. Eventually in the face of disability on the part of an aging family member, you and others in your family, including spouses and children, may find yourselves in the role of primary decision maker for ordinary activities and for those that have more profound implications—such as decisions related to end-of-life situations or to the latter period of life even when the end is not immediately on the horizon.

Shifting the Balance

When the balance of decision-making ability and authority begins to shift, you and your family often face the greatest challenges in decision-making for someone you love but for whom decision-making has always traditionally been the responsibility of that person—usually one or the other parent. Even though in many families discussions about important issues are often framed as joint or collective decisions, the ability of an older person to always disagree with such a decision and refuse to follow remains, even though you and your family find such experiences emotionally difficult and challenging.

With aging and functional and cognitive decline of a loved one, it often becomes necessary for the locus of decision-making authority to shift from the individual to you or another member or members of your family, depending on what arrangements have been made or in which legal jurisdiction the person being cared for and your family reside.

When important decisions are, through necessity, made by you or members of your family or other designated loved ones, the concept of the surrogate decision maker, often also called proxy or power of attorney, comes into play. The role of surrogate is not easy to fulfill, and many people find the task daunting. To ease the task of the surrogate, communication among all those involved is paramount, especially communication throughout your lifetime knowledge of the person for whom surrogacy becomes a necessity.

Some individuals never discuss important personal preferences and wishes with their loved ones. Others are so intent on making sure that everyone dear to them knows what they would want when they can no longer speak for themselves that they discuss it at long length and in great detail. They may even choose to write down their preferences and wishes so that the surrogate has something to form a point of reference should the need arise.

How Decisions Are Made: Personal and Ethical Aspects

When you or a family member is in the position of having to make decisions for a loved one, you or they face a formidable task. Sometimes the transition is easy and everyone seems to know what direction to take. The decision-making however may lead to conflict among you and members of your family or among you, your family, and the health care staff. An understanding of the ethical basis for surrogate decision-making can help elucidate the steps and principles behind the process and also may help you and your family understand why legislation has developed to acknowledge and support the ethical basis of this challenging undertaking.

The essential ethical question in general for cases like that of Maria, Angela, Lisa, and Lorenzo is this: What are the grounds by which a surrogate decision maker, as in this case, a family member, is supposed to act? It is the ethical principle of autonomy that is being challenged in such situations. Normally respecting a person's autonomy allows them to participate in the decision-making process and express their preferences in treatments. A person may accept or refuse a treatment as long as he or she has the mental capacity to make such decisions.

The legal translation of the ethical principle of autonomy is usually reflected in consent-to-treatment legislation, which defines who can make decisions and the basis by which personal health care decisions are made. In keeping with this ethical principle, if a person does not have the mental capacity to express his or her autonomous choices, it falls to a surrogate to do so in their place and on their behalf.

This is where the problem lies. Many family members who undertake the role of surrogate erroneously believe that their decision-making responsibilities are based on what they themselves believe the right decision should be reflecting their values and needs rather than those of the person on whose behalf they are acting. In fact, the measure that determines what a correct decision should be is, whenever possible, not what they want but what they believe the person they are acting for would have wanted had he or she been able to express his or her wishes. The challenge is how would you as a child know what your parent would have wanted in a difficult situation that in all likelihood was never specifically discussed?

Is There a Way to Make Things Clear?

During the past few years, there has been a lot of effort to have people express their wishes for future care should they not be able to participate in the decision, through the development of what are often referred to as *living wills*. The more formal term is *advance directive*.

The idea behind this approach is that a person, by filling out a form, usually with the assistance and participation of a family member, often the one who may end up acting as the surrogate, lays out the framework by which difficult decisions might be made. For example, the person may make it clear on the form that he or she would never want a permanent feeding tube or kidney dialysis or cardiac resuscitation under defined circumstances or maybe never at all. By indicating their choices in a documented fashion with the usual important discussions that should take place, the likelihood is that the surrogate will feel more comfortable making difficult decisions. This is especially important when you or a family member may feel compelled to decline specific treatments based on what you believe your parent would have wanted and had indicated on the advance directive form and during the discussion.

In the case of Maria and her family, in the absence of a formal written document, the question could be raised as to whether Angela was fulfilling her role as surrogate acting on Maria's behalf. It may be that without an advance directive/living will and formal discussions about what she may have wanted, it is somewhat more difficult to know what Maria might have wanted under the circumstances of her last illness.

Specifically, her family agreed that she was not a devout Catholic, so that strong religious principles would not likely be a governing factor in how she might have decided if she could express herself. The comments about her made by Lorenzo suggest that her personal values and view of things would not necessarily support the degree of intervention and extreme positions that Angela was taking. If Lorenzo and Lisa took a strong stand and challenged Angela with their view of what Maria would have wanted, it is likely that ethically and legally the health care team could have refused Angela's demands. However, because the father and sister accepted Angela's leadership, it became difficult for the health care team to turn to other members of the family for guidance. Sometimes families agree to decisions among themselves. They do this to maintain peace in the future rather than undertake conflict that may have long-lasting and destructive effects after the death has occurred. At these times, the family looks back at what transpired and has to come to terms with their decisions.

It might have been worthwhile for the ethicist and one of the trusted team members to have discussed with Angela why she was demanding such extremes of intervention and try to direct her to think about what her mother's values and feelings would likely have been rather than what she wanted to be done. If this did not achieve the goal, the ethical challenge for the health care team would be whether they could justify interventions that they did not feel would be of any value and in fact might cause harm or prolonged suffering in Maria's last days of life.

These are the kinds of difficult challenges that are faced by health care providers as they deal with family members whose views may not clearly reflect what the parent may have wanted. Yet there is no way to ignore those family members' wishes without undermining the fabric of the family structure. After all, it is the family that has to live with their decisions. Whatever they do often takes on a life of its own as part of the family's narrative after the fact, and a story of conflict can be destructive to future family cohesiveness and relationships.

Points to Remember

- It is never easy to make end-of-life decisions on behalf of a loved one.
- Open discussions about wishes and preferences for future decisions can alleviate conflicts in the decision-making process when surrogates are in a position to make such decisions. Though difficult for some families, these discussions are often key to future decisions in difficult situations.
- The test of the decision-making process, as much as possible, should reflect what the surrogate decision maker truly believes the person would have wanted had he or she been able to express his or her wishes. The decision should not be made based on the beliefs and wishes of the surrogate.
- Written documents such as living wills or advance directives can sometimes be of value but only if their content is discussed with those charged with making the decisions so that misinterpretation of the written wishes does not occur.

5

Truth-Telling as an Example of Balancing Benefits and Harms

As I was about to enter the room in my clinic area where the patient was sitting, his wife and eldest son held me back. "What are you going to tell him today?" the son asked. He had accompanied his father, Arnold, a patient with possible Alzheimer's disease, when I first suggested special neuropsychological tests might be useful in confirming the already suspected diagnosis.

The patient's wife had already given a compelling picture of dementia of the Alzheimer type. All the other tests had been consistent with the diagnosis and did not suggest another cause for the patient's repetitiveness, forgetfulness, and loss of higher intellectual capabilities. I had requested the more extensive tests to confirm the diagnosis and to help get the patient moving ahead with treatment. The wife piped in, "Please don't tell him anything terrible today. I do not think he or I could handle it."

The son looked at his mother with the appearance of sympathy but then added, "Mom, we have to tell him because it is getting harder and harder to answer his questions about what is going on."

I led both of them inside my office while my secretary took more information from the patient. "I have to tell him what I believe is going on and what I hope to do in the future," I told them. "It is hard and usually counterproductive to not tell the truth. If I am not honest, I will have squandered his trust in me, and I cannot realistically start him on any therapy for the disease or provide him with any educational materials. Most important for the two of you, we could not discuss or explore future planning because why would he allow it if we said everything was okay?"

I continued, "The fear of the unknown is often worse than the known." I assured them I would frame my comments in the context of hope for the future. This would be critical to the patient's participation in the process, as well as keeping his trust in me, and in them. The wife sighed in agreement, and the son went to get his father.

"So, Arnold, you know I have been concerned along with your wife and son about some of the problems you have been having with your memory and tendency to repeat things," I said. Arnold nodded. "I have the final set of tests I sent you for, which I wanted to do to confirm my suspicions that you have some sort of dementia—a problem with the brain and its ability to remember and do other important things. If you recall, I told you last time that it could be due to a number of causes, such as little strokes or, as it seems to be in your case, Alzheimer's disease, in the early form."

I could see the look of consternation on his face as he focused on my every word. He looked at his wife and son and then back to me. I continued, "I feel strongly enough about the diagnosis that I would like to prescribe one of the newer drugs that have been shown in studies, and I can say in my own patient experience, to be sometimes effective in improving mental function." I continued, "Even if there is no major improvement, the evidence suggests strongly that the medications slow the progress of the disease, which is also important, because you are in its earlier stages." Then I asked him, "What do you think about that prospect of starting a medication to either improve your memory or slow down the progress of the disease?"

He nodded when I suggested the drug treatment. His wife asked about side effects. I outlined the common and important possible side effects. I explained that I usually start with a very low dose and increase it gradually, which usually helps curb side effects, and that most patients I had treated over the years tolerated the drug and many benefited from it. I gave them the prescription and an appointment for a follow-up a few weeks later.

As Arnold left with the prescription in hand, his wife said, "I never thought we could get through this. Thanks." Some weeks later he returned, and it was clear he was tolerating the medication. His family felt that he was more alert and engaged with what was going on around him—something we often see when the medication is beneficial even when formal mental status testing does not show any substantial improvement. Arnold was pleased with the result and said he had no problem continuing with the medication, which is what we decided to do, now in a somewhat higher dose.

As part of the basic underpinnings of family relationships, what is spoken of when it comes to difficult issues may determine how decisions are ultimately made. Families often struggle with just what they should reveal to those they love, as a way of expressing their desire to prevent unnecessary harm and perhaps protect their loved one from a painful truth. The truth when it reflects serious medical conditions may cause fear or a sense of doom in the person receiving the information, which may occur when revealing a diagnosis of Alzheimer's disease or cancer.

I recall in my early days of training when it was common to avoid telling patients that they had cancer, often at the request of the family. This meant that a complex fabric of half-truths and sometimes outright lies were told as tests and treatments were undertaken for reasons that were fabricated to avoid the reality of the condition.

Since those early years of my practice in the late 1960s and early '70s, much has changed in the concepts of communication and the duty to be truthful other than in very unusual and often temporary circumstances. This change is partly because of the need to be honest in order to carry out complex and often difficult chemotherapy and other treatments. In addition is the recognition of our professional and ethical obligations to our patients and their families. Being upfront with patients has an ethical basis in respect for autonomy, even for those with clinical conditions in which mental capacity may be compromised. Unless the person is incapable at any level of understanding a serious diagnosis, most contemporary physicians would concur in telling the truth.

The issue is rarely *what* to tell but rather *how* to tell. Most physicians experienced in the field use a process by which the information and plan of treatment and prognosis is couched in hope so that the person does not feel abandoned and forlorn. This includes the commitment that whatever can be done will be done to assure comfort and avoid symptoms associated with the condition.

The importance of truth-telling in Alzheimer's disease and other serious medical conditions goes beyond good clinical practice in which trust is maintained between the patient and the physician. It has an ethical basis in respect for autonomy, even for those with clinical conditions like Alzheimer's disease in which mental capacity may be partially or seriously compromised.

With the advent of drugs presently available for use in dementia, more patients and their families are seeking help earlier in the course of the disease when a substantial degree of mental capacity may still be in place. The ethical principle of beneficence—that of doing something good for the patient—is another important principle by which telling the truth is warranted. It's difficult to provide a potentially beneficial treatment, which may have side effects that you may want the patient to accept, at least in the short term, without telling them why.

The family's desire to avoid harming the patient is understandable, and in the days before starting potentially effective treatments, this desire may have swayed physicians to avoid telling the whole truth. This approach has little merit in contemporary practice. I have had many family members request I withhold the truth from their loved one with dementia, but after discussion we agree on the truth-telling with the sympathetic support approach, which I have found to be clinically and emotionally beneficial to all concerned.

In the days when we used to obscure the truth when dealing with patients who had cancer, I had an experience that has stayed with me ever since as the result of not having been truthful to a patient at the request of a strong-willed family, many of whom were physicians.

In that case, an elderly woman was found to have metastatic lung cancer of unclear primary source. This was complicated by persistent fluid accumulation between the lung and the rib cage (pleural effusion). She was transferred to the long-term care facility at which I worked for palliative care. As soon as the decision for the transfer was made, the patient's three children approached me. Two of the children, respected physicians, "demanded" that she not be told of her diagnosis. All three concurred. I asked what they wanted her to be told about her diagnosis and the reason for the transfer to the long-term care facility. They said, "Use the term *inflammation*, for which the cause is mysterious and the treatment uncertain. She is from an era when the term *inflammation* was used a lot." I reluctantly agreed, as I had not had much experience in such cases, and the family was adamant in their request.

I instructed the nursing staff and the attending physician to use the term *inflammation* whenever they discussed her clinical condition with her. They were a bit skeptical but agreed to try to be consistent in responding to her questions. Over time, she deteriorated, and the fluid on the lung became increasingly symptomatic, requiring frequent removal of fluid with a needle. Finally, a minor surgical procedure was attempted to decrease the recurrence of the fluid, which provided temporary and only modest relief. A member of the family stayed by the bedside at all times, which decreased the likelihood of any private conversation between the patient and me.

One day, I passed her room and noticed that no family member was with the patient. The patient beckoned me to enter. "Where is your family?" I asked.

"They are all away at my grandson's graduation from medical school today. I am too weak to go." She went on, "Tell me, what is this terrible inflammation that I have? It is so mysterious. There just doesn't seem to be any treatment for it. It is worse than cancer. At least with cancer you know what you are dealing with. With inflammation there just doesn't seem to be any answer. I hope someone is doing research on this inflammation. It is a terrible disease."

She died some time afterward. The family unfortunately never had the opportunity to discuss the realities of her dying or give her the opportunity to reveal her deepest thoughts or to reminisce about the wonderful experiences they had all shared together—a process that many people at the end of their lives find satisfying and affirming of the value of the life they have lived. The family could not bring themselves to discuss the reality of her malignant illness with their mother.

Some years later, I realized that a young post-graduate physician who was working on my team was the grandson of this patient. I revealed to him the conversation I had had with his grandmother. He acknowledged that the family realized too late that they had done his grandmother a terrible disservice by keeping the truth from her, thereby eliminating their ability to tell her things that they would have liked to say. It also prevented her from anticipating and planning a conclusion to her life. The so-called conspiracy of silence resulted in a loss for the last chances of intimacy between the patient's children and herself. It was the last time in my career that I agreed to withhold the truth from a patient.

I have found with reassurance and a gentle, gradual process in revealing the truth—within the context of hope and support—the concerns of the family usually melt away. The physician and patient, with the help of the family, can then develop the therapeutic alliance needed to accept the diagnosis and explore treatment options. Treatment, whether of Alzheimer's disease or the different kinds of cancer, usually includes therapies such as medications, surgery or chemotherapy, and social supports, which in the case of Alzheimer's disease may include day programs. With such diseases, linkages to important support groups such as the Alzheimer's or cancer societies for educational and emotional support are often helpful. The reasons for truth-telling are professionally and ethically sound and should be the approach of the caring and supportive physician who may have to convince the family of the need professionally and ethically to act in a truthful manner.

For a family, it may require a good deal of soul searching and mutual support as well as the willingness to deal with anger and fear as the person you love so much finds out a terrible truth. However, once the truth is out, the basis of trust is established, and the difficult decisions of the necessity of treatments and the implications for everyone can be faced honestly and with the integrity of knowing that anything that has to be discussed can be discussed. It is usually liberating for the patient and for the families to not have to lie. Invariably it becomes impossible to maintain a consistent subterfuge, and, when the truth comes out, an important element of trust may be lost. It is in the nature of such illnesses that trust becomes the most important element of successful treatment.

Points to Remember

- Telling the truth to those you love when their care is at stake is key to developing and maintaining trust.
- It may seem that avoiding the truth might be beneficial if a family member is concerned about inducing fear, dread, and depression in the mind of the loved family member who has a serious diagnosis.
- As part of building a trusting relationship between the patient, family and physician, telling the truth can be instrumental in moving forward with complex treatments and the long-term goals of care.
- It is important to take into account cultural differences as in some situations telling the truth is considered to be potentially dangerous and can be instrumental in bad outcomes. If that is part of the cultural belief-system, it is important for the physician and other health care providers to understand and explain the framework in which they must work while trying to respect cultural values.
- Most physicians in concert with supportive family members understand that how the truth is revealed and couched within a context of hope is at least as important as the very fact of telling the truth.

6

Challenges in Age-Based Medical Care: It Isn't Easy to Be Old and Sick

Considering the number of elderly people in the developed world, one would think that the care of elderly patients, including the specialty of geriatric medicine, and the field of long-term care (nursing home care) would be well developed and sophisticated. Unfortunately, this is not the case, at least in most jurisdictions, although there are places where attempts at improving the system for the care of aged people, especially those who are frail and in great need, are taking place.

Family members of elders are often surprised by some of the negativism they experience when seeking care for an elderly loved one. The response ranges from positive and supportive caring to dismissive with what appears to be a subtext of "blame" for the elder's being sick, needing care, and being a "burden" on the system.

When Samuel Shem's novel, *The House of God,* was published in 1978 depicting life in a modern U.S. hospital, many readers were shocked by the concept of the GOMER (Get Out of My Emergency Room) reflecting the plight of older patients. However, the physicians in training who read the book recognized, even with the hyperbole of the black humor, the veracity of the attitudes reflected in the book, including those toward the old and frail.

In the twenty-first century, with all the education and improvements in care, with the recognition of geriatrics as a medical specialty and its special focus on the elderly, we still read in the papers of *bed blockers:* nursing home patients occupying needed hospital beds while displacing a younger acute care patient who presumably should take precedence over the older person. The terminology used appears to criticize the older patient for getting sick and being in the "wrong" place, as if they want to be in an acute hospital bed rather than somewhere else more suitable to their needs.

Why the Ageism?

In a framework of ethics, the reason ageism must be considered is because the ethical concept of distributive justice attempts to define to whom and for whom are we expected to provide health care services. If there is an inherent reason why the elderly should not qualify for certain health care interventions it should be clear to all, the reasons for this disparity compared to younger individuals. All of us in health care know that there is an element of ageism in the process of decision-making. The challenge is to understand its origins and implications and do our best to dispel faulty reasoning and bias that results in such attitudes.

Why is there such discordance between our purported societal commitments to care for all citizens while many family members experience negative reactions at least sometimes and in some venues when the care of their elderly loved one is in question? Sometimes this apparent "ageism" is blatant, for example, when older people appear to be deprived of ordinary medical treatments because of "age." The problem is that it becomes easy to be cavalier about someone who is ninety-five and seriously ill with statements such as, "They had a good and full life," which on face value may be valid but should not in interfere with good comprehensive medical decision-making.

I witnessed this when my then ninety-four-year-old father, following hip surgery for a fractured hip, fell and hurt his shoulder, to the point that it interfered with his rehabilitation process. The attending physician apparently indicated to one of the rehabilitation staff "that at ninety-four, nothing would be done about the shoulder in any event," which meant proper identification of the injury was made only after insistence by my sister and me. I learned in fact from exploring the literature that some treatments might have been helpful. After discussions, some were undertaken with a modicum of benefit—and without which he could not successfully have undertaken meaningful rehabilitation.

There are probably many explanations for the negative attributes of ageism with all having some part to play in the problem. First is the commonly held belief that we are still a youth-focused culture and society. Even with the number of baby boomers and the redirection of marketing focus to this large population, elderly people are not high on the radar screen. Only those who happen to be elderly themselves or are involved in the care of an older parent or other relative seem to be attuned to the issue.

There continues to be a negative bias in the training of health care professionals, so that relatively few favor aging as an area of special interest. The problems faced by elderly patients do not appear to have the scientific excitement that attracts physicians, nurses, and other health care professionals compared to the subspecialties such as cardiology, neurology, intensive care, and so on. Dealing with dementia and chronic disease does not on the surface sound appealing to many health care professional students, and the experiences they have while training and the modeling and attitudes they witness often work against a desire to enter the field of geriatric care.

On top of this, the payment for looking after elderly people in general is far less than for other fields of medicine. Put all of these together and it is a wonder that anyone enters the field. What it usually means is that at least those of us who focus on geriatric and long-term care have a degree of caring, compassion, and commitment that has drawn us to the field in the face of so many obstacles.

As recently as the summer of 2009 an article in *The New York Times* described the lack of adequate knowledge and understanding for the special challenges that older patients pose to those caring for them. New physicians, entering their post-graduate period, are often woefully unprepared for the realities of a population of geriatric patients, which is a major focus of acute hospitals.

Physician Rosanne M. Leipzig, in her article "The Patients Doctors Don't Know" published on July 2, 2009, notes the following:

> "All medical students are required to have clinical experiences in pediatrics and obstetrics, even though after they graduate most will never treat a child or deliver a baby. Yet there is no requirement for any clinical training in geriatrics, even though patients 65 and older account for 32 percent of the average doctor's workload in surgical care and 43 percent in medical specialty care, and they make up 48 percent of all inpatient hospital days. Medicare, the national health insurance for people 65 and older, contributes more than $8 billion a year to support residency training, yet it does not require that part of that training focus on the unique health care needs of older adults.
>
> "Medicare beneficiaries receive care from doctors who may not have been taught that heart attacks in octogenarians usually present without chest pain, or that confusion can be due to bladder infections, heart attacks or Benadryl. They do not routinely check for memory problems, or know which community resources can help these patients manage their conditions. They're uncomfortable discussing goals of care, and recommend screening tests and treatments to patients who are not going to live long enough to reap the benefits.
>
> "The 2008 Institute of Medicine report "Retooling for an Aging America" resolved that all licensed health care professionals should be required to demonstrate such competence in the care of older adults.

But this resolution lacks teeth. Medical resident training programs that receive Medicare money should be required to demonstrate that their trainees are competent in geriatric care. Medicare should finance medical training in nursing homes. And state licensing and medical specialty boards should require demonstration of geriatric competence for licensing and certification. Basic geriatric knowledge is preventive medicine. Nurses, social workers, pharmacists and other health care professionals should have it, too, in order to improve care for older people. But until doctors get this basic training, we can't even begin to give 80-year-olds the care they need."

Maybe someday these principles will be implemented, but at present this is not generally the case.

In some domains and jurisdictions, things may gradually be changing. In a July 18, 2008, article in *The New York Times*, the subject was the focus on the very old and modern medical treatments that are increasingly offered to and found to be beneficial to elders who in the past were not even considered candidates for such procedures. According to the article, "Data is hard to come by, since people over 75 are scarcely represented in clinical trials, but several geriatricians said that procedures that two decades ago were seldom considered for people in their 90s are now increasingly commonplace. They include hip and knee replacement, cataract surgery, heart valve replacement, bypass operations, pacemaker implantation and treatment for slow-growing cancers that afflict areas like the prostate."

Trying to Assure Good Care

You and your family can help your loved ones by first helping them find a physician who is at least elder friendly and sensitive even if he or she does not have formal training in geriatrics and the care of elderly people. It is always helpful to assist the doctor in the role of trying to care for elderly parents by making sure that necessary information is provided as well as finding ways to be available for any discussions about care planning that may have to be considered. This is time consuming, but it is the only way you can assure quality and continuity of care.

If you have a number of siblings, it is worth figuring out who will do what so as not to overburden any of you. It's also important that a physician have just one primary contact to work with when difficult decisions have to be considered—at times a meeting with you as a family might be in order, but such events have to be planned and organized to make the best use of precious time and human resources.

Most important is that you and your family who will be involved in the caregiving support system must talk to each other and to your loved one about what values and beliefs will have to be considered in future planning. A collective commitment to make sure that your parents' wishes are known and, whenever possible, respected is critical. Discussions as to beliefs and values should take place whenever the opportunity arises. Knowing how to separate your own value systems from those of your parents is important.

It is common to find children making decisions based on their own beliefs about what is valuable in life or in end-of-life care without asking themselves, "What is it that our mother would want" (if she cannot communicate, for example) and why and then consider how to implement those wishes under the given clinical circumstances.

For example, if your parents are and always have been religious, even if you and your siblings are not, the implications of religious values must not be ignored when it comes to end-of-life decisions. Sometimes it is helpful to seek advice from a suitable and compassionate and knowledgeable clergy member to clarify religious principles that may play an important role in how decisions might be made. This is especially important if you and your siblings no longer subscribe to the religious beliefs of your parents or even if you think they are "foolish." The important issue is the respect for your parents and for their autonomy in decision-making especially when they can no longer participate in decisions. This is one of the greatest challenges to children and other family members when they struggle to make a "right" decision and one that they can live with for the rest of their lives without remorse.

Points to Remember

- Caring for an elderly loved one is a major challenge in the current climate of health care in North America. Although recognition of the challenge has increased, families must be vigilant and supportive to achieve their care goals.
- Finding physicians and other health care providers who are friendly toward and knowledgeable about elderly people can help the patient and family achieve their goals.
- Family members should communicate as much as possible to try to determine their loved one's values and wishes so that when the time comes and difficult decisions have to be made, they are in the best position to make such decisions.
- Once the family makes decisions, usually with the help of supportive and knowledgeable health care providers and other advisers, they should accept the decisions and try to avoid the "what ifs" that can often undermine acceptance with a degree of comfort and equanimity.

7

Balancing Acts: When Goals Conflict

Sometimes it is difficult to decide what to do with the various choices in care, especially when the implications of the choices and the goals and values they represent can be diametrically opposed. For example, what if your parent has made it clear before becoming ill that he would not want a feeding tube or even nutritional supplements if he is not able to eat adequately? What if he would not necessarily die from the disease he has, other than the fact that he cannot take in adequate food?

A common example is late-stage Parkinson's disease, in which, in addition to problems with mobility, which interfere with the ability to walk and participate in self-care, there is often a profound problem with swallowing. First the problem is with the process of eating taking a long time. Then it is with the difficulty in eating normal-sized morsels of food, and then with the ability to ingest and swallow sufficient amounts of food to maintain adequate nutrition.

What if your father clearly indicated in the early stages of Parkinson's disease that he would not want a feeding tube or even nutritional supplements (that nowadays come in cans with different flavors and consistencies) if he develops problems with eating and drinking? Now that he has reached that state, you as a child have difficulty accepting his wishes. Despite being conscious and capable of participating in talking and interacting with family and friends, he refuses even nutritional supplements to augment his otherwise meager diet to maintain his nutrition and weight. You find it difficult to fathom that something as simple as an enriched supplement should be rejected when without it the result will be further decline and ultimately death.

Your goals as the child of an aging parent are clearly conflicted. On the one hand, you want to respect your father's wishes and his right to them. But on the other hand, you do not want him to starve to death when something as apparently as simple as a food supplement might provide sufficient nutritional sustenance to allow many more months of life. You understand that a feeding tube would be out of the question and was rejected in principle by him long before he was as ill and immobile as he is at present.

But this seems to be a different challenge—changing the content and makeup of what is being fed to him rather than changing the way it is being provided. What if he said at some point in the past when clearly his decision-making capacity was intact, "If I ever get to the point that I cannot enjoy the ordinary foods that make me happy and need 'unnatural concoctions' to keep me going, it is enough. Let me go." What if the dietician says rather than using a commercial food supplement she can add thickening agents to his usual foods and create "shakes" and other natural recipes that are enriched nutritionally and he rejects them because they are not the normal food that he wants to eat? This is not an easy conundrum to unravel.

Watching a parent "starve" gradually is difficult for any child. But respecting your parent's wishes is a strong motivating force and principle for most children and other loving family members. The challenge then becomes finding the balance between your goals as a child and your wishes to maintain your father alive, and the respect that you feel is owed to him that allows decisions to be made that you do not necessarily agree with.

If there is still an ability to discuss the options, it might be possible to find a compromise. What if you could get your father to agree to a short trial of an enriched diet, but not one using artificial supplements? What if you could frame the trial of supplements in such a way that if, after two to four weeks, he did not like what he was getting even after some time to experiment with different textures and flavors, you would agree to discontinue the process? This way, even though there is an apparent conflict in goals, there might be some scope for agreement and an attempt to bring the goals of each of you into some sort of alignment.

If such a process were possible, a number of benefits accrue. First, there is an attempt to preserve your father's life for a longer period and the no-less-important factor of demonstrating your respect for his participation in the decision-making process. This would be a true reflection of your devotion to him as your parent and as a person whose values count and will not be ignored even if they are at odds with yours and those of other loving family members. If the trial turns out to be successful, you have achieved your goals without undermining his.

As part of the trial of supplements or diet modification, there would have to be the proviso that it could be stopped at any time even if "successful" and if it is not palatable or agreeable. Most important the sense of caring and trying to "do the right thing" is likely to be felt by you and your family. If not successful, you can at least know that you tried to provide care and at the same time provide your father with the respect and reverence he deserves.

Even if his death was perhaps somewhat premature, it was the way he wanted it and that counts for a lot.

Children will pursue very creative ways to fulfill their goals of respect while trying to keep a parent alive! I recall a patient who, while cognitively intact and knowing that she had a progressive neurological disease, instructed her children that in no way did she want a feeding tube for the purposes of providing her with artificial nutrition and hydration. She had reached such a state, and it was clear that she would soon succumb to her illness and the lack of nutrition and hydration.

The son, a pediatrician, asked the medical staff whether they could insert a catheter into her bloodstream so that she could receive nutrients by the intravenous route. He felt that this would not be contrary to her instructions of "no feeding tube" but would allow her to survive a longer period. A review by the hospital ethics consultants concluded that "total parenteral nutrition," which in essence was being asked for, was in fact just another means of providing artificial nutrition and hydration, which the patient rejected in the first place. It would have been unethical to undermine the wishes of the patient by finding an alternative route to provide the same sort of nutritional support. It was rejected by the ethicists as a viable option, and the patient was allowed to succumb to her illnesses without any nutritional intervention.

Points to Remember

- Conflicts in decision-making by caring family members in which a number of choices exist are common.
- There is not always a clearly "right" answer to such ethical and therapeutic conundrums.
- Family members must weigh out and seek an acceptable balance in how decisions are made and make the commitment to live with that decision and accept that there are not always good answers to difficult treatment questions.
- Decisions in feeding are among the most challenging of such end-of-life decisions.

8

The Many Players in Ethics and Care

Sometimes a situation is complicated because of the number of players involved in challenging decisions. At times it is a spouse in conflict with children; other times, siblings are in conflict with each other. With the complicated structure of contemporary families, it may be a conflict between the children, for example, of a first marriage with a subsequent spouse. There are times when the family structure can be complicated, and even if legally there is a clearly designated decision maker, the other players can instigate conflict.

A good example of the degree to which there is conflict, even at times leading to public and media attention, is the Florida case of Terri Schiavo. She was a young woman in what was characterized as a *persistent vegetative state*. Her husband and legal power of attorney had requested that her feeding tube be removed, based on what he had indicated were her wishes as best as he could interpret them. Her parents had no legal authority to make decisions on her part but felt their parental duty to oppose her husband's decision. In this spirit, they mobilized enormous sympathy and support for their position including that of Florida's Governor Jeb Bush. He crafted an individual specific piece of legislation that was passed in Florida that for a period of some months was able to override a court decision that would have allowed the feeding tube to be removed. A higher court ruling later overturned the legislation as being illegal thereby allowing the tube ultimately to be removed.

In this extreme case, there were many players involved in what on the surface might appear to be a relatively clear-cut decision on the part of her husband, who had waited for more than eight years to see if any improvement or hope of recovery might occur. Under normal circumstances, he was Terri's legally determined surrogate decision maker, and in the face of his clear belief that she would not have wanted to be maintained in her present state, the tube would have been removed and she would have been allowed to die. But her family managed to mobilize many advocacy groups who took the position that Terri had a "right to life" that even her husband should not have been allowed to override.

The parents disputed the basis for his decision-making and implied ulterior motives that were not in her best interests. The last attempt to argue in favor of keeping the tube in place took the position that Terri had been a practicing Catholic and that a 2004 *allocution* (a formal or authoritative advisory address) by the Pope was interpreted by those supporting the continuation of the tube feeding, that it would be an abrogation of Catholic religious duties to remove the source of feeding from individuals like Terri. The issue of whether or not she had been a practicing Catholic was raised, which begged the question as what constitutes a person "practicing a religion."

One can see the number of players with different motivations and views that had become involved in one high-profile clinical situation. This in many ways reflects comparable but less dramatic situations all over North America. This case became famous because of the media coverage and the fact that the case became a *cause célèbre* for many interest groups. Similar cases and situations of conflict occur all the time, because the players involved have their own views of the situation and their own values. At times the wishes of the person were not clearly defined or, just as often, ignored because they were not as clearly communicated as might have been desirable.

One way to try to address the needs and desires of the many parties involved in a difficult decision is for you and your family to meet as a group, sometimes with a facilitator (for example, a social worker or ethicist) to try to understand where each of you in the family is coming from. More and more organizations have developed ethics committees and ethicists to help families work through the often conflicting values and wishes that can lead to discord among even the most devoted family members.

The process of review and deliberation with the assistance of an ethicist might help all involved understand why certain decisions have to be made, even when the decision is not what some individual members of a family would prefer. Going through the process, although not guaranteed to find an acceptable "solution," often goes a long way toward helping those involved accept whatever decision is made in a more equitable manner. Sometimes it may not feel like your family has "gotten it right," but at least it is "righter" than it might have been without the important and often-revealing exploratory and deliberative process.

The more players involved, the more challenging is the process. The goal is to reach as acceptable a solution as possible. All family members involved should understand why the decision is being made and accept it as the "best" decision possible under the difficult circumstances that often exist at the end of life.

Points to Remember

- When there are a number of family members involved in end-of-life or other important decision-making, the final decision can be a complex process.
- All the players involved have to understand their roles, legally, morally, and as part of the family unit so that the best decision possible is made.
- The ultimate goal is to try to make the final decision reflect what it is believed that the loved one's views and values would have been and what they would likely choose if they were able to voice their opinion at the time the decision is being made.
- After the decision is made, all the players should do their best to come to terms with the process and the ultimate decision as being the "best" one possible under the circumstances to avoid future persistent conflict, guilt, anger, and other negative feelings.

9

Is Quality of Life Everything? Secular and Religious Views

"I am not sure how my mother would interpret the need to amputate her gangrenous left leg," Nathan, the son, said. Although he had been brought up in a Jewish religious household, he had long since taken a less-observant lifestyle—if anything he had become secular in his views and in many ways had personally rejected many tenets of the religion that was dear to his parents.

His mother, Rose, was eighty-five years old and had diabetes and had a stroke three years previously, which left her unable to speak. Because of her diabetes, she had blood vessel disease that affected the arteries to her brain, which resulted in the stroke, as well as the blood vessels to her legs that resulted in the gangrene. She could not speak but could indicate indirectly answers to specific questions. Rose was still observant in her Jewish tradition before her stroke that led to chronic care hospitalization. Since the leg became gangrenous, her mental state had deteriorated, and it seemed that she was less awake than she had been previously. It was felt that her changed level of responsiveness was likely partially if not predominantly due to the infection in her leg, although damage to her brain from the stroke was also likely.

"I wish I knew the right thing to do," Nathan told me. "I do not want her to die. But I am not sure if having an amputation is something that she would want in order to remain alive, but she is not communicative or able to appreciate those around her who love her."

It was decided to have the son speak to the rabbi of the synagogue that she attended until she became too ill for any advice to be meaningful in terms of treatment options. The rabbi knew her well, and the son felt that perhaps he could provide some insight into what his mother might want to do in keeping with her strong religious beliefs. Nathan wanted to respect his mother's values even though he no longer was particularly involved with his Judaism. He respected the fact that his mother had been observant throughout her life.

The rabbi visited the hospital and tried to speak to Rose who seemed to recognize him through the way her face lit up when she saw him. He asked her about how she felt, but it was difficult to ascertain whether her responses were positive or negative or consistent. The rabbi knew that the hospital tried to accommodate her religious preferences by providing kosher food. The son said they had been good in respecting issues in accordance with what he requested even though beyond the food there was not much more that he could think of. He had no siblings, and his aunts and uncles were old and could not readily visit Rose. He did not feel comfortable turning to them for advice as he was never that close to them during his adult years, even though he had been so as a child and teenager. The last meaningful Jewish tradition he had personally participated in was his own Bar Mitzvah, and he had done that because at the time it seemed there was no alternative to going through with it even though he already felt alienated from the Jewish experience and traditions.

"What is the right thing to do if I want to respect her Judaism, and I cannot determine what her preference is in terms of the amputation?" he questioned. He continued the discussion with the rabbi. "The doctors say she will die without the surgery but can live at least a number of months and maybe a few years depending on other factors and good fortune with the surgery. Because she has had a stroke and is not mobile, having the amputation will not particularly alter her mobility, and she will continue to be dependent on others, but she should be able to sit up and get wheeled around in a wheelchair after surgery. That is the situation at present because of her stroke."

The rabbi said, "According to Jewish Law, tradition, and the underlying tenets of Judaism, unless she is expected to die shortly, our obligation as well as hers is to save her life, even at the expense of losing her leg. This 'saving of a life' is an underlying ethical and religious principle of Judaism, and unless you feel that she has abandoned her beliefs and importance of her religion, that is what she would or should choose to do if keeping her Jewish principles matters. I never spoke to her about such issues on a personal level, but when she attended my evening education classes, we did discuss issues of medicine and Judaism, and she seemed to understand and agree with most of the principles which were discussed, even though clearly they were theoretical, rather than personal."

Nathan acknowledged that he did not notice any change in her commitment to her Jewish values before her stroke that would make him believe that she might not follow those tenets for herself in the current state as expressed by the rabbi.

Nathan went in with the rabbi by his side and said to his mother, "Mom, I just spoke to the rabbi about your leg, which has a terrible infection. The doctors feel that it has to be amputated to save your life. I believe that you would want your life saved if possible. I want to give permission to the doctors. Is that okay?"

The two of them as well as a nurse watched her response, and even though Rose could not speak, it appeared to each of them that she understood the essence of the talk and acknowledged it. Nathan felt that he had enough basis from what the rabbi said and what he was able to glean from his mother's response to agree to the surgery. He felt that the idea of sanctity of life, which was so important in Judaism, was probably what Rose would want. Because he wanted to make the best decision possible on behalf of his mother's likely wishes, he chose to take the action he did.

As it turned out, the surgery went well and without having a gangrenous leg, her mental state improved substantially after the operation. She was able to be up in the wheelchair, and Nathan felt he did the right thing by respecting what he believed to be his mother's values.

Things don't always go as smoothly as the case of Rose and Nathan. Sometimes staff members feel at odds with the decisions made by families, even when they can imagine in some way what values are at stake, but the decisions seem alien to their own values. An example of that kind of struggle is the following case:

Thomas was a man of sixty-eight years who had been in a chronic care hospital for more than twelve years. He had been admitted because of an unusual neurological condition that was progressive and over time interfered with his diaphragm (breathing muscle that separates the abdomen and the chest) as well as his chest wall muscles. He not only had difficulty breathing, but also was having increased difficulty in eating.

Despite all this he was mentally alert and was an active member of the patient advisory committee, sometimes needing help in how he communicated because of his breathing problems. All kinds of technological gadgets had been devised to assist him in his communication abilities and how he got around, which included an electric wheelchair, which he could maneuver reasonably well with the limited use of his right hand that had also been affected by his illness.

He had previously been a fairly devout Catholic but had expressed to the attending physician and some of the nurses on the unit during the past few years as his illness progressed that he was no longer sure that the views of the religion about the sanctity of life and the necessary steps needed to preserve it were as important to him as he realized what the future of his illness had in store for him. Yet when there was an opportunity to celebrate a holiday or be taken to a religious service, he requested to go. He also continued to wear a cross, which had been given to him by his mother when he was an adolescent and had said it had strong sentimental meaning to him.

He had little in the way of living family. One nephew, Phillip, who lived in California, acted as his surrogate and managed to visit about every six months. During those visits Phillip would get updates from his uncle and from the health care staff as to Thomas's progress and prognosis. On one of the visits Thomas told Phillip that he wanted to do a living will—the content of which was fairly simple. It said, "I do not want to be a 'vegetable' and do not want to be kept alive by a permanent feeding tube or permanent respirator. If I reach that point, please respect my quality of life and remove such treatments." A copy of this document signed by Phillip on behalf of Thomas was left on the chart, but none of the staff at the time spoke to Thomas about what he might have meant by terms such as *vegetable*.

Over time, Thomas's condition deteriorated, and he had one episode of pneumonia followed soon after by a second. During each episode his mental state became clouded, and he was not able to communicate using the devices that he had to assist him. But with treatment he improved and once again was able to participate in some of his previous activities, but at a much-reduced level. A point was reached when he had a series of infections and did not make a good recovery. He had a feeding tube inserted because he could not eat. At the time it was believed to be "temporary." It was not clear whether his diaphragmatic respirator device would be sufficient to maintain his respiratory needs; therefore, a discussion about whether a full respirator would be considered was pursued. Phillip was called and when he heard of the deterioration, he said he would arrange to come if he could but then asked, "Haven't we reached the point that my uncle meant when he said he didn't want to be a vegetable and that he did not want a feeding tube?"

The staff held a meeting. Some of the nurses felt strongly that not treating him and removing the feeding tube would be tantamount to "killing." The removal of the feeding tube, they said, was against their professional standards. As practicing Catholics they felt because Thomas was also a Catholic all steps should be taken to keep him alive and that feeding was just part of that normal human commitment. They had to be reminded that their personal values and interpretation of religious views was not applicable to Thomas, who had clearly indicated that the effect of his religious leanings had diminished considerably and that his living will focused more on his quality of life rather than on its sanctity.

The challenge for everyone was trying to interpret what Thomas might have meant by the term *vegetable* and whether his present state would likely be interpreted in lay terms as fulfilling that definition. Everyone could understand that his living will was clear about the feeding tube, which was therefore removed so that the only nutrition being provided was through fluid infusions.

Phillip arrived a few days later, with Thomas in a semi-comatose state. "Even though I did not know my uncle intimately, I believe I understand what he meant by vegetable and how his religious views changed over the past few years. He kept his connection to Catholicism as part of his cultural and historical relationship, having been brought up in a Catholic family, but rejected many of the religious tenets and practices. He stopped attending Mass years ago and celebrated the Christian holidays for their traditions not for their religious implications. He mentioned to me a few times in the last year that his quality of life was what mattered most to him. He told me that if he could not communicate and be part of the activities of the place and enjoy food, which was one of his big joys, he would just as well be allowed to die." Phillip continued, "I think that is what he would want now, and I am prepared to take whatever steps to assure this is what will happen."

Some of the staff mentioned their concern about discontinuing the feeding tube and allowing the respiratory function to decline without resorting to more respiratory assistance. They were reminded that patients or their surrogates legally could always choose to decline therapy as part of respect for their autonomy and the legal framework of consent to treatment, which included informed refusal. They were reminded that it was our professional duty to assist our patients in these personal choices. In this situation, it was clear that Thomas's desire for quality of life rather than any religious-based concept that might include life's sanctity was his to choose, and our professional and ethical duty was to support his decisions.

The next day the feeding tube's function was discontinued, and on Phillip's instructions no antibiotics were given for the next episode of chest infection, which occurred quickly. Thomas was kept comfortable and within a few days he succumbed to his illness. Most of the staff felt that they had respected his wishes, even though a few questioned whether they should have been more assertive in trying to convince Phillip because they could no longer convince Thomas of life's infinite value and that trying to save him again would be the right thing to do. Phillip was certain that he had fulfilled his duty as a caring surrogate and had acted on Thomas's wishes in keeping with his desire for a dignified death that respected his desire for quality of life, even if it meant less of it.

Many of us live in multicultural environments, especially in urban North America. The richness of this mosaic of different ethnic, cultural, and religious affiliations is sometimes counterbalanced in the health care field by tensions and challenges that arise out of different perspectives on the meaning of health care decisions. Sometimes health care professionals fail to appreciate or understand the foundational belief systems that are expressed by family members when decisions are being made. They respond from their own ethnic, cultural, or religious perspective that may lead to conflict and difficulties in providing optimal and sensitive clinical care.

You and your family may be called on to help interpret decisions to health care professionals from a perspective that is different from those providing the care. Depending on the degree of difference, some of your family members may feel that the needs and perspective of your loved one is not being adequately acknowledged or ignored. Sometimes family members may not know enough about the underlying religious values of their loved one to accurately reflect how those values translate into decision-making. Depending on the age differential among the family members who are close to or have been engaged in cultural or religious experiences of the parents, some may feel incapable of reflecting the wishes and values of a parent. Sometimes it requires assistance from a religious leader to help interpret the clinical situation and the treatment options and what the religious expectations might be to help in the struggle to make a decision that is believed to reflect a loved one's religiously based ethical values.

Religious and cultural views must be considered when as family members you are asked to make decisions on behalf of those you love. The translations of these views into the ethical principles that guide your decision-making is the basis of why such views are respected. The challenge is this: even if you do not believe in or support those views, unless there is an overwhelming reason to reject them, your duty is to try to respect them and incorporate them into how you make those difficult end-of-life decisions. In such a way you and your family can incorporate the richness of your family's values and all others in society can do the same so that the many views that members of our society have and how they want to deal with illness and end-of-life issues are respected.

When *Quality of Life* Rather than Religious Issues Are in Question

Brian, a distant friend, called me for advice about his mother. She was living in a nursing home in another city, and Brian would visit every few months. Laura, now ninety-six, had been managing well in her own apartment despite debilitating arthritis, diabetes, and mild Parkinson's disease until just about two years before she finally moved into the nursing home, where she had managed reasonably well for almost a year. Although gradually declining, she continued to function and seemed mentally intact although at times she complained of being lonely.

The call came because Laura had not been well for the previous three days, and Brian was called by his brother Frank who lived in the same city as their mother. Frank had been called by the head nurse of Laura's unit and told that she was declining and that he should come as soon as he could. Frank had been away for a couple of days and had not realized that there was anything wrong. At first the staff felt that it was just a bit of an off day for Laura and that she had not eaten all that much. On the second day nothing on her tray was touched, and she was reluctant to drink much but did get up a bit from bed and took her medications. By the third day she could not get out of bed and became delirious, talking nonsense and not recognizing the staff.

Frank called Brian and said the staff felt that their mother was in the last stages of her life and wanted permission to treat her in a palliative fashion. He could not understand from them what they thought was happening. The doctor said she was "dehydrated" but could not define the underlying cause. Because they could not get tests or provide specific treatment such as intravenous fluids in the nursing home, all he could say was that she seemed to be declining and that he and the staff felt that she should be made comfortable because she had "no quality of life."

Over the phone the two brothers asked me what I thought they should do. Neither of them felt that Laura had indicated to them during their previous visits—Frank less than a week previously and Brian's a month ago—that she had given up on life. If anything she had expressed an interest in seeing her grandchildren and her two new great grandchildren who had been born during the previous year—plans were under way to arrange for those visits to her.

Given that neither brother had any reason to believe that Laura would not want to be given the chance to be evaluated and treated if what she had was potentially reversible, their question of "what to do" was pretty clear. The comments about Laura's "quality of life" that the health care staff expressed appeared to be premature and circular—without treatment clearly she had little quality of life, but with treatment she might improve sufficiently to be able to enjoy important aspects of her life. At that point they did not know what was going on with her clinically.

Being old and sick makes a person look bad, and unless the clinical picture is reasonably clear it can be difficult to know what the treatment options or prognosis might be. By doing nothing, however, the outcome is pretty clear.

The brothers chose to have Laura transferred to the general hospital to at least find out what was wrong with her. Within a few hours it was clear that her condition was beyond repair. She had late-stage kidney and heart failure, and dialysis was not a real option. Further medical treatments might at best postpone her dying for a short period but not allow her to return to any semblance of interactive life.

At that point, Frank and Brian agreed that indeed there was no meaningful quality of life to be offered to Laura. In keeping with what they believed would likely have been her wishes, they instructed the doctors to make her comfortable and allow her to die, which occurred within a few days. They felt, however, that by transferring her to the hospital to know what was going on, they could face each other in comfort. They had done whatever they could do within reason and with respect to Laura when the difficult decisions had to be made.

This situation reminded me of another case I was involved in many years ago, which demonstrated for me how important communication of values and meanings is when discussing decisions that may affect a person's future life and potential treatments.

The patient, Margaret, was sixty years old, had a severe degenerative neurological disorder, the cause of which was a bit of a medical mystery, and had been in a chronic care hospital for many years, with virtually no use of any of her limbs. Through the marvels of technology, she had a gizmo that allowed her to turn the pages of a book that could be placed on a stand so she could read. In addition to books on tape and occasional television, reading was her main source of enjoyment. Margaret generally had a positive and realistic view of her life. She loved meeting medical students, whom I would often take to talk to her, so that she could explain the progress of her disease and how she coped with each stage of it and its progressive disabling effects.

Her daughter, Elizabeth, was a well-known musician who traveled extensively. The patient wanted a meeting about future care decisions as the idea of the living will (advance directive) had come into being. She wanted to express her preferences to her daughter and those who would likely be involved in her care. In the meeting with her daughter and Dr. Lawrence, her primary care doctor, she said she did not want any "heroic" measures or any "tubes" to keep her alive. She wanted to be assured of a "quality of life" even within the framework of her neurological condition, which she had learned to adapt to over the years and which did not interfere with the intellectual and emotional richness of her life. Her wishes were noted in her medical record. The daughter was about to leave on an international overseas tour and left some phone numbers for contact with the nursing staff. This was before the days of cell phones and e-mail.

About two weeks after the meeting I received an urgent call from Dr. Lawrence. Margaret had severe sepsis, likely a result of a urinary tract infection that had gone into her blood system, and she was clearly at risk of dying. Margaret was almost in a stupor and could not comment on possible treatment. Elizabeth was in transit, and a message left at the various hotels for which we had the phone numbers revealed that she would be out on a tour for a number of hours. Dr. Lawrence, a dedicated, thoughtful, and compassionate physician, asked, "What should I do? Margaret had said 'no heroics and no tubes.' I know I could give her intravenous antibiotics and probably save her, but maybe this is not what she would want."

I went with Dr. Lawrence to see Margaret, who clearly was in a severe state, such that without immediate treatment she would probably die in a short while. I spoke to her, but other than some grimaces and gibberish that had no specific meaning, I could not converse meaningfully with her. A urine sample had by chance been sent for routine culture some days previously (because she had a catheter in her bladder so she could pass urine), and this revealed a bacteria and sensitivity to various antibiotics that indicated a good chance that the sepsis was caused by an infection from her bladder and that the germ would normally respond to ordinary antibiotics, which would have to be given intravenously, that is to say by a "tube."

After discussion and soul searching, Dr. Lawrence and I decided to put in an intravenous line and give her antibiotic and fluid therapy. In the meanwhile we left messages at the hotel where her daughter was staying expressing the urgency of our call. Within four hours of starting treatment, Margaret's condition began to improve. By the next morning her fever was down and she was awake, but a bit groggy.

In the night a call had come in from her daughter, and we explained what we did and said that we hoped her mother would pull through but that we had to discuss her wishes for the future the next time she was in town, which she said would be in less than a week.

Within two days, Margaret was almost back to her "old self," and it was felt worthwhile starting the discussion of what had transpired with her even before her daughter was due to arrive three days hence—just in case there was another setback and we were forced to face a similar situation. I entered her room with Dr. Lawrence, whom Margaret was clearly delighted to see by the way her face lit up. After the greetings and introductory comments, Margaret indicated that she was feeling a bit better but could not get back to her routine yet, especially having the ability to concentrate on the book she was reading before her sudden illness.

"I am happy you are feeling better so soon after being so ill. You do understand how ill you were, don't you?" I asked.

She replied, "I don't remember much of the past two days other than feeling pretty punk the other evening when the nurse came in and measured my temperature and then came back again a while after and measured it again. I once had something like this about a year ago when I got the flu, but after I started shivering, I seem to have lost my ability to remember what happened, although I sort of recall you coming to see me with Dr. Lawrence. I do not recall any details until late last night when things seemed to come back to me."

I went on, "You recall the meeting we all had with Elizabeth before she went on her tour, that you did not want any heroics, tubes, and such treatments. Well we were just in that situation the other night. You are deathly ill, and you needed a tube (intravenous) so that antibiotics could be given and some urgent blood tests were required. Because we could not get Elizabeth on the phone because she was overseas to discuss if we should go ahead with what we believed could be life-saving treatment, we decided to do so even though we knew it might result in your being upset with us for intervening and not letting you 'die in peace.' You had mentioned that goal when we had our previous discussion. I hope we did the right thing but feel that we should clarify what your wishes are now and again when your daughter comes back."

She looked at Dr. Lawrence and me with wide eyes, almost tearful, and said, "That kind of treatment is not what I meant by 'heroics'; I meant breathing tubes and machines and feeding tubes because I can no longer eat and the situation would be that I will not become conscious again. You know the kind of 'heroic' things that doctors do to patients rather than letting them die. That is what I want to avoid, not what you did. After all, I haven't finished my book."

She smiled and with her head motioned toward the book on her bedside, which she asked that we put on her book holder and attach the page-turning apparatus. She continued, "When Elizabeth comes back, for sure we have to discuss this again so everyone is clear about what I mean so that the two of you and the other staff understand my wishes for the future."

We had the discussion the following week. Elizabeth was tearful when she realized just how close she was to having lost her mother because she and we had not fully pursued the details of Margaret's wishes. We took the opportunity to do a more in-depth discussion about her wishes, which were put into a written advance directive that outlined certain options in the future for possible treatments.

The main benefit of writing everything down was the discussion we all had that accompanied the probing questions. Even though many people including health care providers feel most comfortable with written documents that outline the limits to future treatments, it appears that the most important aspect of the whole process is for the surrogate decision makers (who are usually family members) along with interested health care providers to understand as clearly as possible what value systems are reflected in the decisions. When those are known, the writing of details becomes less important, as there are always unanticipated twists of fate that may present a clinical situation that was not exactly addressed in a written directive.

Sometimes the family is in great conflict trying to decide how far to go when they hear that their loved one's "quality of life" is not or will not be good, and they are asked to forgo potentially life-saving treatment to avoid putting their loved in a state of poor "quality of life." The problem is, for many people, "quality of life" is hard to define. For one person a life with all kinds of suffering, pain, and limitations may be acceptable; whereas, for another it might not.

The struggle for the family is often how far they should go to determine if there is any potential for treatment when intervention might result in compromised "quality of life" but not doing something dramatic will result in certain death. This is a burdensome responsibility for the surrogate. The challenge for the surrogate is to try to determine what he or she believes the loved one would have wanted under the circumstance. From there one can formulate a plan that tries to address those values while also respecting the advice of those responsible for clinical care.

If you and your family understand the underlying values and principles that your loved one would want respected, it is usually easier intellectually if not emotionally to know when to decide to refuse certain types of treatment. With modern medicine many treatments may be available that are not exactly what people may have been thinking about when they considered possible limits to medical treatments. Family discussions are a low technology interaction, but one that is crucial if patients and families want to avoid some of the high technology medical interventions that may be or become available that perhaps had not even been considered when initial discussions were undertaken.

Points to Remember

- Family members should try to understand the underlying principles behind a loved one's preferences in end-of-life decision-making.
- Strong religious views and values may play an important role in how some individuals would like their end-of-life care to be undertaken.

- It is important for family members to understand that their loved one's religious or secular values, not their own values, should be the basis for such difficult decisions.
- Communicating end-of-life preferences between patients and their loved ones is the critical step in assuring the best of such difficult decisions.
- If a written document is to be used as part of the planning process, the most important aspect of creating such a document is a discussion with those involved as to the meaning of the words and the values expressed within the document so that ambivalent instructions can be avoided.
- Personal values, whether religious or secular, are important as part of what is considered in end-of-life decision-making, and family members and other loved ones should do their best in trying to understand the complexity and meaning of such values and how and when they were expressed.

10

Issues in Feeding and Drinking

Probably no other issue evokes such strong emotional reactions among family members and health care professionals as well as various religious leaders as eating and drinking. One of the fundamental characteristics of all human beings and all societies is the importance of eating and drinking. In all societies, food and drink play a central role in human relationships and activities. We use food and drink in all celebrations, demonstrations of love and devotion, and in all human tragedies. It would be virtually unthinkable to not offer friends and family food and drink when visiting whatever the reason, happy or sad. Virtually all social occasions pivot on the act of eating and drinking. Going "out for a drink" or a "cup of coffee" or "doing lunch" or "coming over for dinner or brunch" are central pieces of all human interactions.

The social attributes of food and drink reflect the basic human need and desire to nourish those we love, from birth until death. One of the first acts of human attachment is breast feeding (suckling) a newborn infant. Whether that mode or another one is chosen during infancy, the bonding process that occurs with feeding may set the stage for many human interactions and relationships throughout a person's lifetime. There are parents and cultures in which the act of preparing food and providing it to one's loved ones has such a central role that stories and humor abound as they relate to the act of feeding and eating. With the growth of multiculturalism many individuals now have available to them foods from all over the world. In most Western urban communities one can eat from a whole range of food types prepared in traditional and sometimes unusual and unfamiliar but often attractive ways.

If there is any problem with the contemporary translation of the primordial quest for providing and receiving food and drink, it is the contemporary excessive consumption of food. Much contemporary food is prepared in a "fast food" manner, which often detracts from any special culinary qualities of the food and is often perceived as less connected to the desire to nourish and nurture than to consume as many calories as possible as quickly as possible. On the surface this seems to contradict the traditional use and meaning of food and drink. It may merely be a contemporary manifestation of the high pressured life lived by many individuals and the ready availability in compressed time periods of easily obtainable and relatively inexpensive nourishment—however limited its palatability, freshness, or nutritional balance.

Most individuals gravitate toward certain foods when they are in particularly stressful situations or when they feel a need to be emotionally nurtured. So-called comfort foods are often items that have had a special meaning or place during the developmental period and may often have positive or significant associations. For example, when ill children are given some type of soup by a loving parent or grandparent, they often form deep positive associations with the flavor and aroma of that soup.

It is not by chance that the popular "Chicken Soup for the Soul" book series has been read by so many individuals of diverse ethnic and cultural backgrounds because of the nurturing symbolism of chicken soup (or any other comparable soup). The nurturing association in the titles of the books attracts readers interested in finding ways to address their emotional needs under various circumstances and periods of their life.

As a young adult traveler, I traipsed all over Copenhagen in search of peanut butter for which I had a hankering I could not explain. When, after a prolonged search, as it was not a food (in the early 1960s) commonly eaten in that country, I found a small jar of it at an exorbitant price, I consumed it at one sitting, virtually right out of the jar.

It is therefore not surprising that in situations of illness and need and especially during end-of-life periods, the importance of food and drink may reach proportions and have real and symbolic meanings beyond what might seem rational to health care providers. This is unless they too experienced as part of their personal lives comparable situations and can project their understanding and feelings to those for whom they are expected to provide professional care and advice. Few other issues raise the importance of ethical decision-making for families more than eating and drinking. It may be related to strong cultural, personal, historical, or powerful religious influences, but any and all of these cannot be ignored by family members and health care providers when such situations arise.

The Meaning of Food and Drink

Julie turned away from her bedridden father and toward the doctor and nurse. "I just don't know what to do," she said quietly. Even though she was a registered nurse working in a pediatric ward and dealt with seriously ill children all the time, this experience when it affected Robert, her father, was difficult for her. Despite being a health care professional and one of two children, Julie's sense of desperation was profound. Many children or spouses of patients hospitalized or living in long-term care facilities all over the world experience these feelings. Her mother, Sophie, and brother Steve, both equally devoted and caring, had agreed to have Julie as the center of communication and decision-making. She was the one who could visit Robert in the hospital most often.

Of all the ethical challenges and heart-rending decisions that families face when their loved ones reach the latter part of life is what happens when they can no longer feed themselves and even with help are not able to get adequate food and drink for sustenance. For families and for health care professionals, the choices can be difficult and the values and implications in terms of love and devotion are often tested more than in any other way that occurs in medical decision-making.

The availability of *artificial nutrition and hydration* (AHN), which is the clinical term that reflects the fact that what is being done is not "natural" but for many individuals seems to be interpreted as the equivalent of the more human terms of food and drink. AHN has made end-of-life care decisions even more difficult for all concerned in the decision-making process. Patients with illnesses that prevent them from ingesting, digesting, or absorbing adequate amounts of food and fluids can now be provided with, via feeding tubes and intravenous infusions, nutrients and water that can sustain them in both short-term and long-term medical situations.

As the provision of food and water even when provided by AHN is often symbolically linked to caring and considered a demonstration of compassion, nurturing, and commitment, some, whether for religious or humanitarian secular reasons, believe there is an obligation to artificially supply nutrition to the sick and dying. Others are of the opinion that artificial nutritional support is a medical treatment not required or appropriate in all situations because of the associated burdens and the possibility that it might compromise what many refer to as quality-of-life issues. AHN is without doubt a controversial issue for many because of the emotional or religious implications of its use.

To continue with the case study, Robert, Julie's eighty-three-year-old father had had a stroke six months earlier and was severely neurologically impaired. Because he was unable to eat, a feeding tube was inserted into his stomach soon after his admission to the hospital. It was hoped this would sustain him while his condition stabilized and he recovered. However, there had been little change in his condition since admission six months previously, and he has had recurrent infections at the feeding tube entry site.

Robert's family was concerned about the pain and discomfort he was experiencing due to these repeated infections. They had hoped he would recover from the stroke, but this has become increasingly unlikely. Robert had told his wife years before when talking about a cousin who had sustained a terrible stroke that he would not want life-sustaining treatment if he were in a condition from which he would not recover and would never be able to eat and talk and enjoy his family. The family is now questioning whether Robert would have wanted to be kept alive in his current state. At a family meeting, Julie, her brother Steve, and their mother, Sophie, voiced concerns to Robert's doctor. The doctor explained to them that discontinuing the use of the feeding tube was an alternative they might wish to consider.

An Emotional Conflict with No Easy Answers

A few years previously, Julie was named as surrogate decision maker for her mother and father. Steve agreed to that designation because he lived out of town. However, neither of the parents had discussed in any detail or wrote advance directives describing the end-of-life care they would prefer should something terrible happen to them. The family is now facing the dilemma of whether the removal of the feeding tube is more than a medical treatment decision because, unlike other medical procedures, it would involve discontinuing the supply of the basic requirements for life—food and fluids even though provided by the technology of AHN rather than through the "natural" means of eating and drinking .

They are also concerned that removing the feeding tube would be equivalent to the criminal act of euthanasia. Sophie wishes there was some way the doctor would make important decisions like this. Steve, Julie's brother who lives in Vancouver, has been to Toronto a couple of times to visit their father since the stroke. He and his mother have deferred most of the decisions about Robert to Julie, because she is a nurse and should understand the medical implications of such a decision. They feel she should know more about such situations to make the decision that is "best for Dad."

The family's first concern that they have already discussed among themselves is whether AHN is a basic need or a medical treatment. They have already broached that subject with the doctor and have tried to find information about opinions on the subject on the Internet. They have discovered that there are lots of different views about the ethical and clinical implications of AHN.

Some of the articles they found considered AHN a basic need and not an actual medical treatment. If the family subscribed to this view, they might feel obligated to provide nutrition and fluids—withdrawal of the feeding tube would not be an option. On further exploration they discovered that the issue is a source of controversy even among health care professionals, ethicists, and religious scholars.

Julie is conflicted. She has had to face similar situations with some of the sick children she has cared for over the years. For Julie, despite her professional experience, the challenge of dealing with her father makes it extremely difficult because it is so personal and everyone in the family is looking to her for leadership.

Their quest for information made them realize that there is no clear universal consensus on this issue. A number of scholarly groups that have carefully studied and deliberated the issue, including the Canadian Special Senate Committee on Euthanasia and Assisted Suicide and the British Medical Association, while recognizing the perceived difference between AHN and other treatments, have concluded it is a medical treatment.

Despite such a conclusion that they found through their Internet searches, Robert's family is also worried about the idea of withdrawing a life-sustaining treatment they've already started. Julie's mother is particularly concerned that, by removing the feeding tube or discontinuing its use, she is in essence abandoning her husband in his time of need. She wonders whether the act of withdrawing treatment could be construed as euthanasia—something she rejects in principle and has done so when cases have been discussed in the media.

They discovered through exploring the commentaries available through the Internet that many of the ethics scholars indicate that, while the withdrawing of treatment may be psychologically or emotionally more difficult than withholding treatment, there is no moral difference between the two actions. This ethical view is supported by common law, which recognizes that medical treatment can be withheld or withdrawn based on the wishes of the patient or family if they are the designated surrogates, even if it leads to death. The Canadian Medical Association commentary on the issue distinguishes between euthanasia, which in Canada is illegal, and the withholding and withdrawing of unwanted, inappropriate, or futile medical treatment, which is not illegal.

The Ethical Debate: Balancing the Principles

Along with the establishment that AHN is a medical treatment and the believed moral equivalence of refusing, withholding, and withdrawal of medical treatments, the ethical principles of autonomy and beneficence become the overriding factors in this decision-making process. It is helpful for Julie as the main decision maker to understand this as she struggles with her decision on behalf of the family and her father.

The ethical principle of autonomy requires that informed decisions made by competent patients, or their substitute decision makers, be respected. This ethical principle is supported legally by Health Care Consent Acts in most common-law (English-speaking countries) jurisdictions. It requires patients or their decision maker, in this situation Julie, to consent to or refuse medical treatments before they are performed. As artificial nutrition is considered a medical treatment, it can be accepted or refused by the patient or substitute decision maker. The family went through that struggle when they agreed to have the tube put in with the hope that Robert would recover, which unfortunately did not occur. Now, the use of the tube could legally and ethically be discontinued in view of the fact that his recovery has not been what everyone had hoped for.

Due to his medical condition, Robert is no longer able to directly express his wishes regarding his care. Julie, his appointed substitute decision maker, has to make the difficult decision for him. Fortunately, he had the foresight to appoint Julie who in many ways has the greatest breadth of understanding of the issues, but that did not make the decision easy for her.

Depending on where a person lives, if a substitute is not appointed, there are various rules as to who in the family would be asked to make such difficult decisions. In some jurisdictions, one has to go through the legal system to get permission to make such difficult decisions, which just adds another layer of complexity to what is already a difficult and emotionally challenging process. The fact that Robert had previously appointed her has made it easier for everyone in the family to let her struggle with the decision and—finally after conferring with them as important family members—make the final decision.

The Process of Decision-Making

As the decision maker, Julie would have the obligation to follow any advance directive outlining her father's wishes that he may have previously made. However, as Robert has not written one, she is expected to make a substituted judgment decision in accord with either verbally expressed wishes or the values he expressed throughout his life or specifically to others. Julie and other family members believe these were expressed during a conversation with Sophie when he said he did not want to be maintained on life-sustaining interventions if he were in a condition from which he would not recover. No one but Sophie was there for the specific conversation. Soon after, during a family visit, she communicated that conversation with Julie and Steve, and it became the basis of their understanding of Robert's wishes should such a circumstance as the present one arise. Julie never specifically asked Robert about what he said, but she assumed her mother's rendition was accurate.

If no one had any idea of Robert's desires or if no agreement could be reached as to Robert's wishes, Julie would have been required to make a *best interests* decision. This is one in which a plan of care generally thought to advance the patient's *best interests* would have been followed. In addition to autonomy, the ethical principle of beneficence imposes a duty on health care professionals to help and to benefit and protect all under their care. Although Robert's wife Sophie feels the doctor should make the decision regarding his care, the physician must respect the wishes of the patient or Julie as the designated decision maker because Robert is no longer able to express his wishes directly.

In cases regarding the withholding or withdrawing of treatment such as AHN, the health care professional's commitment to beneficence is demonstrated by providing the patient and family with appropriate and current clinical information on the usefulness of artificial nutrition and hydration. It also should include aiding the patient and family in weighing the possible benefits and harms of treatment. In addition, for an informed decision to be made, the goals of AHN must be considered in light of the patient's current medical situation.

There might be some benefits to this treatment such as prolonged survival, preservation of muscle and skin integrity, reversal of malnutrition and dehydration, and enhanced healing or stabilization of disease. There are also associated burdens such as irritation, infection or discomfort at the site of tube, aspiration into lungs and potential pneumonia, need to restrain patients to prevent tube pulling, fluid overload resulting in shortness of breath, need for suctioning, fluid retention in the legs as well as disruptions in urinary output and/or incontinence. Depending on the patient's condition and desired medical outcome, AHN may or may not be the best treatment option.

After serious consideration, Julie, representing Robert's family, decided, in keeping with his wishes and in light of his medical prognosis, to discontinue the use of his feeding tube. It was an emotional struggle. She felt the decision to do what he would have wanted if he could have expressed it. The family stayed with him after the tube feeding was discontinued. Over the following five days, he slipped further and further into coma. The staff was wonderful in how they cared for him and how they supported the family with their difficult decision. Steve managed to arrive two days before his father died and was there to support his mother and sister. At the end, they knew they did the right thing and could live with the decision that they made.

In some situations even a written advance directive does not assist in the decision of what to do with late-stage nutrition and hydration. In one such situation, the father had written what had seemed to be a very detailed advance directive stating preferences to not have feeding tubes or even antibiotics if the situation was such that the person was either "terminal" or had a condition with cognitive impairment from which he was not likely to recover. When the clinical situation had deteriorated to the point where a feeding tube was likely to be required for his nutrition to be maintained, the son indicated that since he was there at the time the advance directive was written, he felt that his father did not mean to withhold artificial feeding under the circumstances of his current state of illness.

This resulted in a good deal of controversy as to the meaning of the stipulations in the advance directive and how it impacted on the current state of affairs. Because of the extreme contention in the situation, the matter went to court, which ultimately deferred to the son's interpretation of his father's words at the time they were written.

The conclusion among the staff was that advance directives cannot be depended upon to direct late-stage treatments unless the person makes sure the substitute decision maker clearly understands the meaning of the directions. It's also important that the decision maker not have a conflict of interest or be in an emotional state where they may find it difficult to implement the wishes. Whenever possible the terms used in the directive should be clearly defined (for example, *terminal* means the following ...). Also, perhaps the patient's physician should be there to interpret the implications of any decisions about treatments that are stipulated so that the document is clear and that there is someone else to refer to should there be a conflict with the substitute decision maker's interpretation of the written document.

Points to Remember

- Eating and drinking are core activities for all of us.
- When normal eating and drinking are no longer possible, AHN might have to be considered.
- It is never easy to decide whether or not to provide AHN.
- The process of the decision maker, especially when it is a substitute, must be based on the best estimate of what the person would have wanted had they been able to state their preference—or at least their personal values.
- Even though not putting in a feeding tube is considered ethically equivalent to withdrawing its use, psychologically it feels very

different. Many families have difficulty with the latter decision and equate it with killing their loved one.
- The most important part of the decision-making process is the deliberation and consideration that is given to this difficult decision and the commitment to accept it as the best one possible, once it is made.

When Feeding by Mouth Is the Right Choice— Even if Dangerous

Sometimes the scenario is the flip side of the ones just discussed. A family may struggle to avoid putting in the feeding tube in the first place as a way of providing the last pleasures of life to a loved one—even at the risk that adequate nutrition may not be provided.

The phone message sounded frantic. It was the daughter of Mrs. D, a patient I had been following for more than six years. The daughter was an accountant. She said that her mother was in a nearby general hospital where she had been admitted a few days earlier with pneumonia. The daughter was told by the dietician and speech-language pathologist who had done a swallowing assessment that her mother needed a feeding tube. I left a message for the daughter to call and in the meanwhile reviewed her mother's office chart.

I had seen the patient first because the family physician had some concerns about the diagnosis of dementia and wanted help in assisting the devoted daughter in planning for the future. It appeared that the family physician felt that the daughter's expectations and planning were unrealistic because she wanted to keep her mother at home, with whatever support services were required, rather than have her admitted to a long-term care facility. After my evaluation, I too thought the plans were likely to fail. But I indicated to the daughter that everything reasonable that could be done to fulfill her wishes would be attempted. But I cautioned that much of the caregiving would fall on her and whomever she could hire to provide assistance while she was at work at her busy accounting practice.

Over the years, I was amazed and impressed at how successful the daughter was in keeping her mother at home with a quality of care that was enviable. She found devoted caregivers. From my experience with these caregivers when they accompanied the patient and her daughter to the office, they were completely devoted to the well-being of their patient. I discovered that one of the caregivers was a foreign-trained physician who could not achieve licensure in Canada but was so devoted to the care of the elderly that she chose to be a personal care worker as a way of using her experience and clinical skills. Whenever a medical event occurred, such as infection or an osteoporotic fracture, all appropriate interventions and consultations were arranged without need for hospitalization—a most remarkable feat.

There had been some problems with feeding and swallowing over time. But the caregivers had found ways of preparing food and carefully feeding the patient so that she ate safely and had put on weight and then maintained it. Now, the daughter was in a panic. Not only did her mother require hospitalization for pneumonia, but the speech-language pathologist told her that the risk of recurrent aspiration pneumonia from feeding her mother was so great that she would recommend to the nursing staff that no oral feeds were to be provided. She told the daughter that the only intervention that she could professionally recommend was a permanent feeding tube.

The position taken by the speech-language pathologist reminded me of the first course I took in clinical ethics, soon after I undertook the position of chair of Baycrest Centre's ethics committee in 1994. Because I felt that I had no formal training in ethics, I enrolled in the well-respected Georgetown University one-week intensive course in medical ethics, designed for people like me.

In one of the seminars, a case was presented for discussion by our group, which matched the situation that Mrs. D's daughter described to me. In that case, the speech-language pathologist who participated in the seminar took the position of not feeding a patient with a swallowing disorder because she could cause the patient harm and claimed that her autonomy as a professional was being undermined by the request for oral feeding. The group's discussion focused on the fiduciary responsibility of health care professionals and their professional duty to respect the wishes of competent patients or their designated surrogates even when harm might result.

All seminar members agreed that at times such decisions were difficult. They concluded that, unless it was believed that the decision was not made in a competent manner or that a surrogate decision maker did not understand, appreciate, and accept the inherent risks, their professional obligation was to provide the best care possible while respecting the patient's or surrogate's informed decision and expressed wishes.

Mrs. D's daughter was determined to try to have her mother fed again, after she recovered from her pneumonia, before considering the option of a permanent feeding tube. She said with great fervor that one of the few remaining joys in her mother's life came from eating. She had wonderful and dedicated caregivers who were willing to try to feed her again, especially if they received some professional supervision to avoid aspiration risks. She felt that a feeding tube would be unacceptable to her mother. If that was the only alternative, she would have to consider long and hard as to whether a life with a feeding tube would be what her mother would want. As a devoted surrogate, she felt that she should be given the chance to take the risk to feed her mother.

I spoke to the attending physician, a well-trained geriatrician. He concurred that it was probably premature to assume that a feeding tube was the only option available to the patient. It was agreed that the treatment for the pneumonia should be completed for a few more days. After that, if the situation allowed, gradual reintroduction of feeding initiated by the caregivers already known to the patient, with some supervision by the nurses and speech-language pathologist, would take place.

The patient was discharged home a few days later with plans for a home visit by a community-service swallowing team to assist the caregivers in methods to feed Mrs. D as safely as possible. It worked and she remained at home being carefully fed with no serious problems until she died almost a year later from another unrelated heart condition.

My sister and I experienced a comparable situation with our father who had been hospitalized for a respiratory tract infection. Following a rough few days in the hospital he appeared to have aspirated some food and developed severe respiratory symptoms. The physician, without actually communicating his thoughts to us, ordered that no food be provided to our father until a swallowing study was arranged. We were led to believe it would be within a day or two. In the meanwhile he received only fluids by a needle in his vein.

After two days, we were told that the swallowing study had to be postponed until after a weekend, which was coming up because of staffing and holiday issues. Meanwhile a bronchoscopy (looking down into his lungs with a special telescope) was undertaken by a chest specialist. All the while our father indicated that he was very hungry and wanted to eat. He was alert and understood what had been going on. The bronchoscopy did not indicate anything serious in the lungs or bronchi. When we asked the attending physician who had ordered the swallowing study why we had to wait, he said, "If there is a swallowing problem, we may have to put a permanent feeding tube into your father."

My sister and I were shocked. We knew from previous discussions with my father that in no uncertain terms he had rejected the idea of a permanent feeding tube as a way to provide him with nutrition. The scenario had been formulated by the physician without discussion with the surrogate decision makers or my father, who at the time was able to participate in decisions. We told the physician that what he proposed was unacceptable and that we would start feeding my father if he would not order resumption of meals from the hospital dietary staff.

My sister provided a few meals of yogurt with mixed fruit, and our father managed them very well. We agreed to have him discharged without the swallowing assessment. Two weeks later on a return visit to see my father, I was pleased to photograph him eating some of my wife's special baking "dunked" in milk, which was one of my father's favorite treats. He has managed for more than three years since that event eating and drinking quite adequately, even if slowly.

Framing the Ethical and Emotional Challenge

The ethical and personal family challenge posed by this case is one often faced by families and health care professionals. What do families do when the professionals they depend on make recommendations that they might disagree with? What are the limits to health care professionalism when it comes to respecting competent choices by patients or their surrogates even when the choices pose some risk?

The driving force behind health care professionals' not wanting to participate in treatments that they do not believe in or that might cause harm arise from their professional and ethical principle of beneficence—their deep-seated desire to do good things for their patients. Coupled with this principle is that of nonmaleficence, the commitment to not cause harm. The latter dictum is a powerful force among physicians, as the Hippocratic Oath makes a specific reference to it.

In the face of these compelling professionally ethical principles, when they collide with valid feelings on the part of families, tensions often rise. When there is a conflict between the concept of autonomy, which is what allows patients and surrogates to make informed choices, even when the results may be harmful, and the concept of beneficence or nonmaleficence on the part of health care providers, there is often a sense of conflict.

In the past, health care professionals determined, in most cases, the course of medical treatments. It is now accepted in North American medical practice that patients and surrogates can manifest their autonomy even when the choices may result in treatments and potential outcomes that are in conflict with medical knowledge, opinions, and standard recommendations.

Even though most health care providers understand these tensions, it is important that they do not become cavalier in accepting harmful choices by patients and surrogates. Health care professionals must use their skills and positions of trust to help patients by carefully and patiently explaining why it is that certain recommendations for treatment are made.

Health care professionals possess a powerful instrument they can use to convince patients and their surrogates to consider a treatment. That powerful instrument is their position as a caring, dedicated, and trustworthy professional. Open dialogue, patience, time, and the projection of caring and trust can go a long way in helping patients accept controversial treatments that are recommended by these dedicated professionals.

It is also sometimes worthwhile to agree to discontinue a recommended treatment after a mutually agreed-to time period if the goals of the recommended treatment are not achieved. Sometimes this method allows for a trial of a controversial therapy without having to accept it on a permanent basis. Although it is sometimes psychologically more difficult to discontinue a treatment than to initiate it, without such an option, some potentially beneficial treatments will never be attempted.

It would be sad to think that someone you love might not be offered a trial of tube feeding that could potentially be effective if it could not be stopped once started and shown not to be useful. At the time of initiation of a trial of therapy such as a feeding tube, you and everyone in your family and all the professionals involved should attempt to define the goals that will determine if the treatment will continue or not. It is then somewhat easier for a treatment to be stopped without the staff or you and your family feeling that all of you have caused an unacceptable harm. In essence the harm would have occurred had the feeding tube not been attempted.

Ethical dilemmas around feeding can be challenging. Food is considered by all cultures as an essential component of life. Even though there is much literature disputing or confirming the nature of artificial feeding (through tubes, for example), for many health care professionals, and surrogate decision makers, the prospect of withholding food, even when through a feeding tube, can be a daunting task. Professionals should state their own values or biases when assisting families in the task of decision-making, as there is no way to ignore personal guiding principles when difficult decisions are made.

If a physician, nurse, speech-language pathologist, or nutritionist cannot help patients and their surrogates because of strong personal feelings or values, it is worth requesting assistance from other staff members or from an ethics committee to assist in the decision-making process. For example, if a physician subscribes to a religion in which it is felt that artificial feeding is deemed to be a duty and obligation, that value should be communicated to the family. Then the family will not misconstrue recommendations to insert a tube to be based purely on clinical evidence, but rather on the physician's personal values that may be playing a role.

Another conundrum that I have experienced is exemplified by a case of a gentleman in a chronic care unit of a long-term care hospital. He had sustained a stroke and had a moderate degree of dementia but was still able to take some nourishment by mouth—but not enough to maintain his fluid status, which was supplemented by a twenty-four-hour-a-day subcutaneous (under the skin) infusion of fluids. This caused some discomfort to the patient, but the son, the only family member, accepted this as the price to pay to maintain his father's life, which he was not prepared to forfeit at this point.

A family meeting was held as the health care team was concerned that the amount of supplemental fluids infused was leading to discomfort at the sites where the fluid went in as well as repeated local infections. The son rejected the notion of a feeding tube because he felt his father would not have wanted one. But most importantly he felt that his father could still enjoy taking food by mouth, especially items such as ice cream, which he loved all his life.

"I can't imagine depriving him of one of the last aspects of joy in his life, which would occur if the tube was inserted," the son said. "I think we have to just go on as is and deal with the discomfort."

We then told the son that if he would allow a feeding tube to be inserted, we could provide most of the nutrition and hydration through the tube and thereby eliminate the subcutaneous fluids and still allow his father to have his favorite foods such as ice cream by mouth, thereby allowing him that same degree of enjoyment. The son was not aware of that option but said he would consider it as a compromise.

As we have seen from the cases discussed here, there are often no clear answers in ethical challenges in health care, especially as they pertain to eating and drinking or artificial nutrition and hydration at the latter stages of life. It is important that all health care providers and the families looking after their loved ones recognize the process of deliberation and the examination of values and options. Clear and mutually supportive communication is as important as the ethical principles themselves, when difficult decisions have to be made.

Points to Remember

- It is sometimes reasonable to take chances when it comes to feeding as well as other difficult treatment decisions.
- Make sure all the options are explored and the relative risks and benefits are identified before making a feeding choice.
- When possible, frame the choice and intervention in such a way that if the decision proves to not be effective it can be altered with the least amount of emotional and ethical anguish.
- Sometimes it is possible to hedge one's choice, as when a feeding tube might be required for the bulk of nutrition but the person can still take some elements of food by mouth so as to enjoy texture and flavor, thereby meeting what might appear to be disparate goals.

11

Levels of Care: Finding a Balance Between Giving and Receiving Care

Many caregiving and ethical challenges occur when there is apparent conflict between what health care professionals and family members feel is the right care under the circumstance. The following exemplifies the type of conflict that may occur even among well-meaning people.

"I want my father to be transferred to a general hospital so that all possible care can be provided." These words came from a daughter, the youngest of three siblings. "In addition, while waiting for the transfer, my father should be resuscitated if he has a cardiac arrest," she continued, as her two older brothers sat next to her. The brothers tended to be more passive than their younger sister when health care decisions were being made for their eighty-six-year-old father, who had many severe and complex medical problems.

The father had been on a heavy care continuing care unit (equivalent of a skilled nursing unit in the United States) for just over six months, having been admitted following a number of strokes. He was left non-communicative in addition to having great difficulty with eating and clearing his secretions. He also suffered from severe heart problems, very poor circulation to his feet, and poorly controlled diabetes which caused infections in his feet, with incipient gangrene.

A year before his admission to the continuing care unit/skilled nursing unit, while in another hospital's cardiac care unit because of a heart attack, he had experienced a cardiac arrest due to an irregular heart beat while the daughter was visiting him in his room. He had been successfully resuscitated, although he lost even more of his ability to communicate. Since that time, she had become anxious about his care and arranged for private nursing staff so that he always had someone in the room with him, "just in case." He had continued to deteriorate since that time and had a number of serious infections, each one of which left him weaker and more debilitated and less able to interact with his family or the staff.

The nurses on the unit felt uncomfortable about how much the daughter hovered and questioned their actions. The physician and the team had several meetings with the daughter. They tried to help her understand her father's dismal prognosis, while at the same time assuring her all reasonable care would be provided with a primary focus on his comfort. The daughter consistently rejected any suggestion of limiting treatment, even though her brothers tried to temper her demands. She refused a suggestion made during one of his bouts of pneumonia that he be deemed a palliative care patient with the focus of care being comfort measures only. She became incensed at the suggestion and threatened the staff with legal action if they did not take all steps to treat every medical event fully.

The response of the staff depended on how they viewed her demands. Some felt she should be able to do what she thought was best for her father based on her role as designated surrogate. Others, including the physician, could not believe how far she was prepared to go to get her way. Some nurses felt intimidated by her because she was constantly scrutinizing their actions, either by her presence on the unit or by having her private duty nurse report back to her each action taken by the nursing and other staff.

She was frequently short-tempered with the staff and had even expressed a willingness to make complaints about misconduct to their professional credentialing organizations, having already made a number of complaints to their administrative supervisors. Many of the staff felt that she did not value their caring and competence and some became reluctant to take her father on as a patient because that meant dealing with her. This presented challenges to the head nurse when assignments were being given out.

Not only did the nurses have problems but also the physician expressed frustration. The physician suggested the daughter had gone beyond the usual boundaries of a caring relative and was now undermining the staff's commitment to care and the staff's desire to be responsive to her demands.

The medical situation at hand was another bout of probable aspiration pneumonia. The patient had already had a number of these episodes. All had been treated successfully on the ward of the continuing care hospital. The treatment had not been complex or onerous. The patient was given antibiotics, fluid replacement, and oxygen therapy and suctioning as required. These treatments were provided to many other similar patients on the unit, and the staff felt comfortable providing such a level of care. Moreover, they were concerned, based on previous experiences with many other patients, that even a few days in a general hospital often meant that the patient came back, perhaps with the pneumonia treated, but with other problems such as skin ulcers, especially if there was a long wait in an emergency room due to a shortage of beds or any other delay in admission to a hospital ward.

The staff felt his condition had deteriorated since the last bout of pneumonia, which had occurred only a month earlier. His recovery was even less robust than on previous occasions, and they could see him gradually slipping away physically, with ever-increasing needs for nursing care. Everyone was aware he was at high risk for aspiration and further pneumonia due to his previous strokes. The daughter had categorically refused a feeding tube. Although the staff acknowledged that a feeding tube would not prevent aspiration, the difficulty he had with choking while eating his pureed meals and supplements just added to his problems. The daughter indicated that she understood it would not eliminate the possibility of future episodes of aspiration pneumonia, even though it might provide some benefit, as he clearly had difficulty swallowing—despite special protocols and care by the nurses while feeding him.

When asked what she thought her father would have wanted, she claimed he would have wanted to be kept alive at any cost. She was not able to explain how she knew that and then added, "I want to keep him alive for as long as possible. After all he has been through in his life, he deserves to be kept on this earth for as long as possible no matter what."

Her brothers did not seem as convinced as she was. They admitted to the social worker they did not want interfamily conflict and were prepared to go along with her decisions. She had often taken the leadership and dominant role in family decisions, and they felt it was appropriate that, as the oldest sibling who had been most involved and responsible for care, she be allowed to make the final decisions, even if they might be extreme.

The physician said she did not feel a transfer to a general hospital was warranted and might result in less attentive care than would be provided in the institution that had looked after him for so long. She also noted that with recurrent aspiration pneumonia, the prognosis was not good, and it would be preferable for him to be with people who knew him well and cared for him, so that, should he succumb to his illness, he would be in the company of friends. Finally, the doctor believed, but did not express this concern openly, that a transfer was an inappropriate use of resources because all the patient's care needs could be met well and appropriately on-site and sending him to an acute care hospital was unnecessary. She also believed that the acute care hospital might well send him back with instructions for care rather than admitting him, which could be distressing for the patient and his family.

Exploring the Ethical Issues: Who Makes the Choices of Treatment, and Why

The ethical issues in this case include the role of the surrogate in decision-making and the basis of surrogate decisions. In this situation, it appears there was no clear and compelling indication what the patient would have wanted—for personal or religious reasons, for example—to have all available treatments provided to him.

If the best interests test would be applied to his case, it might well be considered that heroic treatments such a CPR would be inappropriate in view of his multiple medical problems and the gradual and persistent decline in his functional status. In such circumstances, CPR is rarely effective even in the immediate resuscitative attempts, much less long-term survival. Frail elders like this patient have poor outcomes with CPR, according to many studies, even when full resuscitative teams are immediately available.

The issue of whether sending him to a general hospital was a good use of available resources is known as resource allocation and reflects the ethical principle of distributive justice. This ethical principle is often a bit more difficult to decipher, as physicians should generally avoid making allocation judgments on their individual patients.

It would be better if there were institutional policies that clearly defined when and for whom CPR or repeated treatments with antibiotics or transfers to general hospitals would be a fair and reasonable use of the collective resources that exist for such cases. For example, a policy that defined the circumstances under which CPR would or would not be provided and the rationale might take some of the pressure off the staff that felt that the intervention offered little potential benefit and might even be a complete misuse of time and effort. It is they after all who would be called to administer CPR. Many, under the circumstances, might interpret such actions tantamount to assault on this poor dying man. Some staff members had expressed that feeling to the social worker and later on to the ethicist who was called to help explore the situation with the family and the staff.

There are often no clear answers or processes by which complex situations such as this can be satisfactorily unraveled. But clearly understood ethical principles and discussions that allow the staff and the family to go through the process of deliberation might allow all those involved in the final decision to more readily achieve the reasonable and acceptable goals. The goals are, first, to provide care for the patient in a sensitive, humane, and clinically appropriate fashion. Next is to find the best ways to support the family in this time of great challenge and crisis.

Often, with enough patience and discussion, a reasonable common ground can be reached so that after everything is over, the family, especially the daughter, does not feel that she abandoned her father during his time of greatest need and that she and her brothers can agree that they did the right thing for him.

Because of the daughter's reluctance to accept any measure of limits on the care provided to her father, even in the face of his imminent decline, the organization's ethicist was asked to meet with the family and team to help resolve what appeared to be an impending crisis of confidence by the daughter in the staff's competence and dedication to her father. Gradually, after a number of discussions, it was agreed that small incremental steps of palliative-type symptomatic care would be taken to see if the father would respond in any way. When this proved to be the case in terms of his comfort, the daughter reluctantly agreed to a full palliative approach to care, in which the focus was comfort. This proved to be successful, and the father succumbed gradually rather than suddenly with a cardiac arrest so the issue of CPR disappeared from the decision-making process.

Points to Remember

- It is always challenging to decide on any limits to potentially beneficial care in modern medicine.
- Surrogates should try to figure out and whenever possible incorporate what they think their loved one would have wanted when end-of-life decisions are being contemplated.
- When there is a clear conflict between the health care staff and family members, external assistance, often from a clinical ethicist, might help define the problems and the possible options in a less adversarial manner.
- It is important for the health care staff to carefully explain the process of and implications of procedures such as CPR to avoid families requesting such an intervention because of lack of proper information about its benefits and effect on frail elderly individuals.

12

Challenges Posed by the Acute Hospital System

With all the television shows that focus on the dramatic aspects of hospitals and with substantial media attention to hospitals, many people have strong beliefs about what acute hospitals are supposed to do when someone gets sick. The assumption we generally share is that hospitals are places you go when you need urgent or specialized help and that everyone there is dedicated to helping you get better.

The public loves hospital stories, as reflected in the popularity of hospital-based television shows as well as the scores of fictional and nonfictional books on the subject. This is testimony to the intrigue and awe that most people hold about hospitals and the doctors and nurses that make them run.

Yet you and your family, like many people, may not have had a wide range of personal experience with various aspects of the health care system—the acute hospital and its emergency room, in particular.

The challenge for children of elders who enter the acute care system is to make sure they understand and help their parents understand the options that exist for the many major medical decisions they may face. You and your family may assume that everything that should happen in the acute care system has a sound clinical basis. Generally most of us also tend to believe that the clinicians responsible for delivering such care in most circumstances are cognizant of and have internalized the ethical basis for decision-making.

Professionals often struggle with the clinical and ethical decisions as do families. The question for family members should be, "How do we make sure we are doing the right thing, in the face of the common uncertainties that abound in medical decisions?" It may be difficult for you and your family members to accept the reality that things don't always go the way you hope or wish even when the best efforts are made.

How to Say "Yes" to Treatments

Most people assume that, when they enter a hospital, they have in a sense agreed to the general care being offered. In elective situations—that is, when the treatment has been planned in advance, such as with many types of surgery—you generally expect explanations from the doctor before the hospital admission so you know what will be done and why and what might be expected, including some statement of the potential risks of the treatment. This process is formally called *consent to treatment*.

Most people focus primarily on the potential benefits of the proposed treatment ("I should be able to walk pain free after my diseased arthritic hip is replaced by an artificial hip."). You may not focus on potentially catastrophic outcomes (for example, the surgery may not help your hip or you might have problems with the surgery or the hospitalization itself). You often don't think about the prospect of having a stroke during surgery and never being able to walk or speak again, much less think about what happens if the rare and unexpected happens and death ensues. In the same way, even though we all know that driving can be dangerous and people get into accidents and die on the road, most of us do not think about that as we rush to our jobs and pick up our children in good weather and bad.

Because of this tendency to disregard the possibility of adverse outcomes to treatments, the health care profession in keeping with respect for the ethical principle of autonomy has been required to more formally make sure that patients understand the potential benefits and risks of any offered procedure and formally agree to them. This *consent to treatment is* generally laid out formally now in most medical settings. No treatment can be provided by health care professionals without in some way making sure the person either understands and agrees to the general principles of treatment and signs a document stating that the specifics of a certain treatment have been explained and that they agree to have it performed.

Therefore, there are different standards and processes of assuming or getting consent for a specific treatment (such as a surgical procedure) or a series of treatments as part of an ongoing process of care, such as the treatments involved in caring for someone with pneumonia—x-rays, blood tests, intravenous or oral antibiotics, treatment for other conditions that might be made worse by pneumonia such as diabetes that might require changes in treatment or heart failure that might need an alteration of drugs.

Sometimes the hospital may require a special consent to treatment form to be signed. In many other situations, the fact that a person is admitted to the hospital and participates in all care activities is deemed sufficient to demonstrate implied consent, yet some hospitals request a signed acknowledgment that all ordinary treatments necessary for care will be accepted. For the most part, physicians and nurses usually, in addition to the formal process of providing information and confirming agreement to treatments in writing, will explain and explore the possibilities and options whenever there is a substantial change in condition or in the need for changes in treatments,

In urgent and emergency situations, the consent to treatment process may be somewhat different, and the ethical basis for treatment decisions shifts from the respect for *autonomy*, which is reflected in the formal or informal consent process (with the patient or surrogate if he or she is not capable of making decisions), to that of *beneficence*, which means the health care staff try to do what is best under urgent circumstances for the patient until it is possible to figure out what is necessary for the future.

So if someone you love arrives in an emergency room having had a stroke, even in the absence of anyone to give direction to care, all efforts will usually be made to provide treatment to save the person's life irrespective of the circumstances. But at the same time, the health care providers will try to find someone appropriate to provide consent to treatment and give further direction to the approach to care decisions. The avoidance of unnecessary harm, an important ethical commitment as well (*nonmaleficence*), will usually be taken into account. If it is clear or likely that a treatment not only will not be successful but also will result in probable suffering by the patient, the decision might be to not undertake it rather than upset the balance of trying to do good while avoiding harm.

In urgent situations in which the patient cannot be involved in the decisions because cognitive impairment already exists (for example, sepsis in a person with severe dementia), the surrogate is ultimately responsible for the decision. If a surrogate is not available during the period of crisis, the likelihood is that the physicians and nurses will undertake necessary treatments until full discussions can take place with the surrogate decision maker. This means that sometimes potentially invasive and immediately life-saving treatments might be started that are unlikely to fulfill long-term treatment goals. One example would be putting someone on a respirator who is unlikely to survive but whose life can be prolonged by the respirator and other supportive care. Further in-depth discussions and decisions by the surrogates as to when and how to continue or discontinue the treatment would have to follow after the initial life-saving decision is made.

Some individuals and their families try to avoid being in a position of not knowing how to deal with such unexpected outcomes of either planned medical care or urgent care due to a catastrophic illness. They undertake discussions and sometimes fill out a formal advance directive or living will. Although not a panacea for all the possible problems that might occur, the process does give families the solace that they at least discussed the possible issues with their loved ones so that they could respect what they can interpret from the document or discussion when it comes to making difficult decisions.

Knowing that you have discussed your options with your loved ones, when difficult decisions might have to be made, gives you the sense of having made the right decision, if the time comes. This is especially important in the face of difficult choices and differences of professional and sometimes family opinions.

My sister and I experienced this process with my father, aged eighty-nine at the time, who collapsed suddenly in a hospital outpatient clinic waiting for a hearing aid assessment. He had a long-standing history of angina and a previous heart attack but had been stable and taking his medications for many years. He had limited exercise tolerance because of his angina (chest pain), but he was good at taking his nitroglycerin before he walked or after a meal to improve his symptoms.

Before this event by a few years, about a year after the death of our mother, I had a chance to speak to my father on an autumn walk on the boardwalk in Brighton Beach in Brooklyn, where he was still living. I told him how difficult it was to make the decisions we made about discontinuing treatment for our mother and his wife of more than fifty years. He started shedding tears as he listened to my telling him that if possible I wanted to know what he would want if he could not make a decision so that my sister and I could try to make the right decisions for him should a similar situation unfortunately occur.

First of all his response was, "I know I can trust you and Diti to make the right decisions for me."

Because I knew that he would have difficulty expressing himself about details, I continued, "Daddy, it is a bit beyond us making the right decisions for you and of course we know that you trust us. We need to know as well as we can what matters most to you." I continued, "As I know you for this many years, I think I have a pretty good sense of what you would and would not want, should something terrible happen to you and you were not able to express your wishes."

He nodded and I continued, "I think that if what happened to mommy for example or something in the same way happened to you and there would be no hope of your recovering so that you could speak, eat, interact in a meaningful way with us and your grandchildren, that you would prefer that we would not try to keep you alive."

He looked at me as we continued to walk and said, "Yes."

I then continued, "I think for you the quality of your life depends on some degree of your own independence, the ability to read (he has been a devoted *New York Times* reader for as long as I have known him) and speak and laugh and eat. If these things are no longer possible and not likely to be so in the future, you would prefer to be allowed to die."

His response was, "Exactly."

So our end-of-life discussion was over, and I felt satisfied that I understood his wishes and values. That night I told my sister on the phone what we had talked about.

Some years later he had the sudden collapse in the hearing aid clinic in a Chicago hospital. I was on a trip with my family in Quebec. I heard from my sister that after the collapse in the hearing clinic, he was brought immediately to the emergency room, where he was found to have an extremely slow heart rate. First it was thought that all he needed was a pacemaker, which was inserted the next day, following an explanation by me to him about what a safe and excellent treatment that was.

But by the day after, even though his heart was now beating at the normal rate, it was suspected that he had had a small heart attack, and it was recommended that he have an angiogram to see if he needed any special cardiac treatment or surgery. The thought at the time was an angioplasty (widening of the heart's blood vessels with a balloon inserted within them) might be necessary. I spoke to the cardiologist who felt that this was the most likely scenario, but he would not know for sure until after the test.

I spoke to my sister, and we agreed to encourage my father to undergo the procedure. We thought that if they found he needed bypass surgery, he might refuse, and we would support him in that decision because of the potential risks to function including a stroke as a result of the surgery.

The phone rang a few hours later, and it was the cardiologist, who was standing in my father's room saying, "Your father needs urgent bypass surgery. He has a critical block of his left main stem artery (the main one supplying the heart muscle), and if we do not do this soon, he is at high risk of a fatal heart attack." I asked when surgery might be, and he said, "We would like to do it tomorrow. I have booked him but he wants to talk to you and your sister first. She is here right now."

I spoke to my sister, and she confirmed what was going on and said our father was hesitant about the surgery. I told her that even though we had previously decided that he should be able to refuse the surgery if he wanted to, after I heard the report by the cardiologist, I decided to try to impress on him the necessity and urgency of the decision.

I got on the phone with him, "Daddy, the cardiologist feels that you need the bypass surgery urgently. They want to do it tomorrow."

My father said, "Let me think about it."

I replied, "Sure, you have ten seconds, nine, eight, and seven."

He said, "What's the hurry?"

I replied, "The cardiologist is concerned that if we do not do this tomorrow, you may not be around to consider it again."

My father paused for a few seconds and said, "Okay."

I told my sister to go ahead and told my family that we were leaving the next day a bit earlier than initially planned for our drive back to Toronto. From there I would fly to Chicago and would arrive the day after his operation. I was at the same time worried but optimistic that my father had the wherewithal to do well despite his age.

I arrived the day after surgery. He was still in the cardiac surgery intensive care unit and was awake but had lots of tubes coming out of many orifices but was already breathing on his own. He had been taken off the respirator a few hours before my arrival.

As a geriatric specialist, I was worried about his mental state and any signs of confusion after such a major operation with a long anesthetic. But he immediately recognized me and seemed to make sense in all his comments. By the next day all but one of the tubes was removed and he was clear headed and *kibitzing* with the nurses. A cardiac surgeon covering the weekend explained to me the procedure and indicated that all went well during the surgery and that my father was recovering well.

By the following day, he was transferred to a regular medical ward and soon after to a cardiac rehabilitation unit from which he was discharged home a few weeks later.

Even though this scenario went well for my father, my sister, and me, we had to be prepared for the worst, if he had not responded well to the surgery or if there were major complications. At the time I wondered if I had been too precipitous in urging my father to have the surgery without much time to ponder the implications.

Some weeks later, I was struck by the realization that we had made the correct choice when I heard that the father of someone close to us, of a similar age, died while waiting in the hospital for cardiac bypass surgery, which had been booked three days hence. He had asked for a short postponement for a family event—it brought home the reality that sometimes urgent decisions can mean the difference between a good outcome and a tragic one.

We were prepared to deal with the possibility of a bad outcome, and I discovered later that my father had said to my sister before his surgery, "If this does not work out well, let me go." This was in keeping with what he had indicated to me some years earlier in our talk on the Brighton Beach boardwalk about his values when it came to end-of-life care.

How to Say "No" to Treatments

One of the greatest challenges that you as a child of an aging parent and your other family members might face is when you have to decide against treatments that are recommended and that may make the difference between life and death, or between good function and dismal function.

The question and challenge for children is how to maintain the respect you and your siblings have for your parent's decision-making abilities and deal with the reality of their desire to refuse treatments even if the result is contrary to what you and your siblings would want them to do. Even more difficult is when the parent is not able to fully participate in the decision and the children acting as surrogates are faced with the prospect of refusing treatment as they try to act in keeping with their parent's previously expressed wishes or clearly defined value systems.

Preparing for saying "no" is a long process, which usually occurs before the event, which is often the culmination of preceding events or experiences. A fairly common example of individuals deciding to discontinue life-maintaining treatment is often seen within the framework of chronic renal (kidney) failure and long-term dialysis. Even when the treatments are fulfilling their clinical goals and the patient is getting a great deal of psycho-social support, it is not uncommon for such patients to decide to discontinue the dialysis because of what they consider to be a poor quality of life and the burden of continuous attendance at the dialysis unit even knowing that it will mean their death within a few weeks.

Children understandably often struggle with such a decision, especially when things seem to be going relatively well from the clinical viewpoint. They may try to convince their parent to continue with the treatment. Frequently they search frantically for a preferential way to get a kidney transplant, for which it is known that the waiting list is long, sometimes apparently endless, and the wait ultimately fruitless.

I recall a case of an elderly woman who reluctantly agreed to dialysis even though her initial reaction to its possibility was negative. She agreed to try it for three months but in fact continued with it for a number of years. Although she did well, she did complain about the traveling and the time involved in the procedure. As she got older, even though she was managing well clinically, she began to express an existential view that she had lived a long life and could not see a reason to continue.

She was examined to make sure she was not depressed. After that was excluded, within a few weeks she decided that she did not want to participate anymore and opted for a palliative care approach to her final days. This was done and within ten days she succumbed to her illness, comfortable in her decision and in the way she died. She did not have a lot of family with whom to discuss her decision. She did express clearly to her few friends and to the staff that looked after her that this was the right decision for her, and they supported her emotionally as her wish was carried out.

Sometimes such decisions are made in the acute care setting and in an urgent or emergency situation, when there may not be much time for children to consider the decisions of their elderly parents. Often because of uncertainty by the children, decisions are made to undertake major medical treatments that have substantial risks, rather than to refuse treatment based on an understanding of a parent's wishes, if they are unable to communicate because of the illness. The decision can go either way, depending on the understanding that the children have of their parent's previously expressed wishes or values and the potential for the proposed emergency treatment to result in success rather than further disability or suffering.

The difficulty all family members have with saying "no" to potentially life-saving care is the fear that, if the treatment is not tried, their parent for whom they want only the best will die. But if they say "yes" but the outcome is not good, it may result in suffering and the need to withdraw a treatment or medical life support system (such as feeding tubes and respirators), which can be psychologically difficult for a loving family.

Many of the ethical conflicts that occur in general hospitals occur in intensive care units because patients have ended up on respirators and require total care for conditions that were treated in the hope of successful outcome. Now with hope gone, health care staff in the intensive care unit usually request that the life-support treatment be discontinued.

This is often a heart-wrenching experience for the families, but often as well for the staff, especially if they have been involved with the patient over a period of time. For the children it often feels as if they are killing their parent when they agree to stop a respirator or discontinue tube feeding. Even though they may understand intellectually that what they are doing is not killing, but rather letting their parent die from the underlying illness that the technology is not able to reverse, the emotional conflict can be great. Moreover, in some religions, the stopping of life-support systems can be deemed as killing, whereas not initiating treatment can sometimes be more readily justified.

In a contemporary case in Canada that received worldwide media coverage, an elderly orthodox Jewish man had been put on a respirator as part of his treatment for an acute infection, a complication of a multitude of other medical conditions. After a prolonged period of various treatments, removal from the ventilator was attempted, but he could not breathe on his own. When the medical staff came to a decision to discontinue the ventilator treatment, a court order was obtained to stop them from doing so. In this case the family was not able to say "no" to further medical treatment even in the face of unlikely future benefit.

For months while awaiting a definitive legal opinion, the family and the physicians and other health care professional staff and the hospital and many stakeholders became involved in the case. Some bystanders accused the hospital and doctors of attempting to commit euthanasia. Members of the family and other religious leaders suggested the act was in conflict with the concepts of religious freedom. Some doctors resigned from their positions in the intensive care unit while others volunteered to continue treatments.

Ultimately the patient died of natural causes and the case was never reviewed in court—opening the issue up for another similar case, which is likely to occur at some time in the future. How such ethical and legal conundrums are to be avoided is not an easy task. Value systems and the running of the health care system are involved in all such complex situations and decisions.

An important way of dealing with the emotionally charged situation of saying "no" to further treatments—the result of which might result in death of a parent or withdrawing a treatment already in place that is not likely to result in recovery—is to constantly think of what your parent would say to the treatment. This projection of thought back to the parent rather than focusing on your own thoughts and feelings has to become the basis for the decision.

If there were conversations about such possibilities or comments made relevant to another person in a comparable situation in which the parent clearly expressed values, "Please, children, don't ever let that happen to me," when a neighbor's wife, for example, was on respirator life support after a devastating stroke, you might extrapolate what the decision would be if your parent could make it on his or her own.

Trying to draw on your parent's values and beliefs is an important way of preparing for the pain in making such difficult decisions. The thought that the undue suffering will cease and the decision is what you believe your parent would want should provide sufficient solace to allow you to make the decision with the sense that it is right.

Points to Remember

- General hospitals are complex organizations. The stress of an admission for an acute problem or for a pre-arranged treatment can be daunting, especially to an older person and their family.

- Many decisions about treatments occur in acute care hospitals. Sometimes they are about the original illness being treated and sometimes because of events that occurred after the initial treatment.
- Having an idea as to what preferences your loved one likely had about certain situations might be helpful in agreeing to proposed treatments or refusing them.
- Before agreeing to any treatment, get the best explanation possible as to the likely risks and benefits from the person most senior or that you trust most in the care pyramid—that is often the attending or treating physician.
- If things do not work out well after agreement to treatment has been made, it is always possible to refuse further treatments or withdraw some treatments that have already been instituted.
- Withholding and withdrawing potentially life-maintaining or life-sustaining treatments is always difficult but can be the right thing to do if you and your family feel that it is the choice your loved one would have taken under the circumstances.

13

Cardiopulmonary Resuscitation (CPR): Reality and Myth

"Code blue, code blue. 4 west, code blue, code blue, 4 west," announced the overhead speakers.

Doctors stopped what they were doing and started running down the corridors, a red crash cart pushed by two nurses careened around the corridor and arrived at the open door. Two doctors were pressing on the patient's chest while a nurse was pressing a respirator bag attached to a mask over the patient's face.

"What is the rhythm?" a young doctor dressed in a green operating room suit asked.

"V- fib!" the nurse shot back, taping the leads from the monitor onto the patient, who could barely be seen under the group of doctors and nurses.

"Shock him," the doctor ordered as everyone pulled back from the patient as the paddles were applied.

The camera zoomed in on the monitor, which went from chaos to order. A common story line on television medical shows—so common that a study done on the way cardiopulmonary resuscitation was presented on television medical shows was the topic of an article published in *The New England Journal of Medicine* in 1996. In it, 75 percent of the patients survived the immediate arrest, and 67 percent appeared to have survived to hospital discharge—with the reality in clinical practice being perhaps a tenth of that percentage in all ages and closer to 1 percent or less in frail elderly people, especially those living in long-term care facilities. It is the media depiction of CPR that is in most people's minds when the issue of CPR comes up for discussion for their elderly loved one.

With these facts in mind, it is not surprising that of the many controversial issues that recur in the care of older individuals especially those in either acute care hospitals or long-term care facilities CPR is high on the list. Most individuals' knowledge of CPR is limited to the rare personal experience with a friend or family member or as noted already with what is seen in the media. Because in the media depictions of CPR a large portion of those undergoing resuscitation survive, usually with no significant negative result, the thought of not trying to bring a parent "back to life" seems to be an awful and immoral decision to many family members. The struggle to forgo the attempted treatment with what is called a *DNR (do not resuscitate) order* is not easy for many family members. Some scholars have tried to change the designation to *DNAR (do not attempt resuscitation)* to remind us that it is the undertaking of the process of CPR that we are trying to prohibit. However *DNR* is what is generally used in the medical literature and in hospitals in the English-speaking world.

CPR when first described some decades ago was a monumental discovery that changed the practice of medicine. CPR as we recognize it today consists of pumping on the chest in a rhythmic fashion, while providing support in breathing and then providing a variety of treatments including electrically shocking the heart and giving medications to stimulate the heart's function. Before CPR, the only way to stimulate the heart if it ceased to pump was to open the chest cavity (as a surgeon does for an operation on the lungs or heart) and squeeze the heart itself in a rhythmic fashion while finding ways to support respirations (breathing) and correcting what was wrong with the heart that made it stop. This type of treatment was rarely successful, but when it was, it was usually within the context of surgery so that everything was in place for what was a potentially life-saving surgical treatment, through which the heart could be manually compressed to sustain the circulation.

I recall as a second-year medical student coming back to Brooklyn for a summer and working at a local general hospital. It was before the development of CPR as we currently know it. A very ill patient who had problems with his lungs was being assisted as was common in those days by being surrounded from his waist up in an "oxygen tent"—an enclosed hood made of plastic into which oxygen in high concentrations was being provided. In some ways although it increased the amount of oxygen the patient breathed, it cut the person off from many aspects of care and socialization because everyone was afraid to open the tent and allow the oxygen to leak out.

One morning in the middle of ward rounds there was a shout from a nurse, "Mr. so and so in bed 4, he's blue, come quick." Within minutes the bed was surrounded by doctors, the tent was thrown aside, and he was being examined urgently. Moments later an anesthetist and surgeon arrived, and I watched astounded as the patient had a tube put down his throat into his trachea while the surgeon made one long cut through his chest wall, as one would do for a lung operation. He then inserted a gloved hand inside and started squeezing his heart. The bed and floor were covered in blood. After many minutes of squeezing and breathing and looking and listening and monitoring the patient's heart, it was clear that he had died. For days after, despite repeated scrubbings, I felt the tackiness of the spilled blood on the floor around the bed.

With the advent of what was first called closed chest CPR, the procedure could be provided almost anywhere with varying degrees of success depending on the clinical situation. Gradually many people in addition to health care professionals learned to do CPR so it became available almost anywhere. There are few medical interventions as dramatic as someone having a cardiac arrest, often as the result of an accident or electrocution, and see them resuscitated by a passerby or ambulance personnel or police or firemen all of whom are trained to provide CPR. However, the circumstances of those successful outcomes of CPR are usually different from what exists in hospital situations with older patients and especially in nursing homes, where the average age of residents is high and the complexity and degree of underlying medical problems and subsequent physical and mental disabilities enormous.

During my years of medical training, much of which took place in Scotland, CPR was not yet part of local medical practice. It had just been developed a few years before my finishing medical school in 1966 and had been implemented across North America when I undertook my first hospital training placement in Boston in 1967. My experience with it during my year in Boston was less than stellar, as most of the patients seemed to die after what appeared to be heroic efforts on the part of the physicians and nurses involved.

On occasion, especially in the unique environment of the cardiac care unit, a patient survived CPR, usually because their "arrest" was in the context of a known underlying heart condition. They were not only in the best place you could be for the CPR to take place, but the whole event was either anticipated or "witnessed." This meant that effective treatment could be immediately applied. Most important, most of the patients in whom there was any success were not very elderly.

I continued with my medical training in Canada in 1968. During the year after my internship I was in a hospital in Montreal as a medical resident, which had an aggressive CPR commitment. This included a team, which was responsible for all CPR undertakings throughout the hospital. We were as well trained as anyone could be, and the supervisor of the CPR enterprise was dedicated to its success. What I experienced that year was that it was almost impossible for anyone to die in the hospital without an attempt at resuscitation. This was before it was legally permissible to have a do not resuscitate (DNR) order. So whenever someone was found without a pulse or blood pressure, irrespective of the cause of this event, the team was called and CPR was administered until such time as it became clear that it would not be successful.

At the outset of my rotation on the cardiology service where I became a member of the CPR team, I was excited to be able to participate in the most dramatic and exciting kind of care, coupled with the unbridled enthusiasm and almost religious dedication of the medical resident who was the champion of the CPR program. However, over a number of months that I participated in the team, I began to wonder at the wisdom of attempting CPR under circumstances in which I believed that what had happened was death and not a cardiac arrest.

This observation sensitized me to a professional and research interest in CPR eventually among the elderly, whether in hospitals or in nursing homes. My conclusions after many years of observations and review of the studies that had been reported in medical journals is that there are few circumstances where there is justification for providing CPR in elderly frail individuals who suffer from a multitude of underlying medical conditions, whether they are in a general hospital or in a nursing home or other long-term care facility.

For the latter living situation, the overwhelming evidence is even less supportive of benefits from CPR because the circumstances that are required for admission to a nursing home in many ways result in the frailest individuals entering these facilities. Invariably they have many medical conditions, including diabetes, high blood pressure, heart disease, and stroke, as well as substantial degrees of dementia, such as occurs with Alzheimer's disease. With this population, what usually occurs is not a true cardiac arrest, whereby the heart stops for an unusual circumstance that can be reversed by medical treatment (CPR). Most of the true successes in CPR occur in otherwise relatively healthy people who have the wherewithal of surviving CPR and returning to normal function.

Rather, in the frail elderly, especially those who require long-term care to meet their multiple care needs, what happens is death, which includes the heart stopping, but in such a way that attempts to restart it are, in essence, futile.

This means that the underlying conditions that resulted in its stoppage cannot be reversed. Over the years many studies have shown that in the nursing home/long-term care elderly population especially, benefit from CPR with a return to normal function is rare indeed. The result is that many individuals are exposed to the most undignified process of CPR as their last experience in life, when the outcomes are universally dismal. Many of the staff working in nursing homes/long-term care facilities are aware of the awful outcomes of CPR but feel compelled to provide it because many residents (if they are able to express themselves) and many family members feel an obligation to "bring their mother back to life" rather than just accepting that when death occurs, it is final.

The best way to avoid the anguish of having to deal with such a situation is to discuss the possibilities with your loved one long in advance of the need for a nursing home. If there is agreement on the wishes and direction that your parent would prefer related to CPR and other difficult situations, it might be a good idea to do a living will with your parent to define those areas where there is certainty about treatments such as CPR. If this is done, it would allow a DNR order to be written at the time of admission to a nursing home thereby avoiding inappropriate and ineffective attempts at CPR by the staff of the nursing home or at a general hospital if an illness requires transfer to one. If the beliefs are clear and instructions or values are communicated to family members but a written document is not completed, it is still possible for surrogates (often the children) to indicate to the staff of the nursing home that CPR should not be performed and a DNR written on behalf of the parent.

Sometimes, despite the best of efforts, CPR is undertaken when it should not be, and systems need to be developed with proper communication to make sure this does not happen. One case I recall involved an elderly woman who lived in a nursing home. Her only family was a grandson who lived in the same city but rarely saw her. He was notified by the home that his grandmother had been failing lately. She had told him some months earlier, after learning that she had a bowel malignancy, that she did not want more tests and that she should "just be left to be." He had indicated her wishes to the staff at the nursing home but failed to request a DNR order and no one on staff had raised the issue. They had assumed that she would just die in the nursing home from her underlying disease.

One weekend when there were some part-time staff covering the floor, she became mentally confused and had been noted to not be eating or drinking. She was sent to the local emergency room (ER) where she was found on admission to be unresponsive. In the ER, with only a short note from the nursing home's nurse, who admittedly did not know the patient well, she was in the process of undergoing the evaluation to figure out her problems. She could not communicate and was clearly dehydrated. The grandson was out of town and could not be reached by the nursing home or the emergency room doctor at the time of her transfer and admission.

While under emergency room care the patient experienced a cardiac arrest. In the absence of a DNR order and a full history of her condition, CPR was undertaken, which when proven ineffective was discontinued after a period of ten minutes. When the grandson called some hours later, he was dismayed that his grandmother experienced what he felt was an unnecessary indignity but realized eventually that part of it was due to his failure to fully communicate with the staff and their failure to communicate with the emergency room.

To avoid unnecessary and likely ineffectual CPR attempts on their residents, some nursing homes have implemented policies in which the default position is DNR. This means that a resident or family has to formally request that CPR be performed in the event of a cardiac arrest if they wish it attempted. For many families this arrangement is easier to deal with as they do not feel that they have to make an active decision to deprive their parent of a treatment, however apparently futile it might seem to be.

Some nursing homes have recognized the reluctance of many families to provide DNR orders to limit attempts at CPR to those individuals who meet strict criteria that reflect the minimal requirements which are necessary for CPR to have even the remotest chance of success—that the event be witnessed by a member of staff and that it be unexpected. This means that it was not the final likely outcome of a serious illness such as a serious infection, stroke, or other condition. To deal with these situations they have developed policies that stipulate that even in the absence of a DNR order, resuscitation will not be provided unless the event is at least witnessed and unexpected.

With such a policy, most residents of nursing homes do not receive CPR even when a DNR order does not exist. The most common scenario is for a resident of a nursing home to be found without a pulse and blood pressure or breathing, which would imply death has already occurred. CPR does not ever bring people back to life. The *R* in CPR stands for *resuscitation* and not resurrection—which is a point that many family members do not fully understand. In few unusual circumstances if the event is witnessed and truly unexpected, CPR can take place. For those children who are reluctant to request a DNR order, for personal or religious reasons for example, if the nursing home has a comprehensive policy on CPR, with clearly thorough protocols and guidelines that define potential candidates, the likelihood is that it will not be performed without some remote semblance of potential benefit.

Ultimately it must be decided by individuals themselves. This technological marvel was never designed for the frail elderly population. CPR should not be used on them. It does not retrieve them from death. Families may rather accept that a gentle and dignified death may be the best thing at this point that life has to offer. For the children of elderly nursing home residents struggling with such choices, making one that feels right and is ethically and clinically defensible makes clinical and emotional sense.

Points to Remember

- CPR is a dramatic and on occasion life-saving intervention that is rarely effective in the very elderly and frail population.
- For CPR to be effective it must be performed under optimal circumstances: the arrest is witnessed and unexpected and CPR undertaken within moments.
- A do not resuscitate order is the most effective way within the institutional setting to avoid the possibility of ineffective and unwanted CPR. The intent of the DNR order must be communicated by family members to staff members and properly documented.
- If a DNR order exists for an individual in a nursing home/long-term care facility, that information should accompany the individual if they are transferred to another facility such as an acute care hospital.
- Failure to provide CPR should not be misconstrued by concerned family members as a sign of abandoning their loved one or allowing them to die when an alternative might have existed. Rather, it avoids the last moments of life being surrounded by an ineffective and undignified medical intervention that should in most instances be avoided.

14

Long-Term Care

The term *long-term care* has been interpreted in various ways by those involved in the system—often decrying what they believe to be inappropriate or a too narrow use of the term. The concept reflects the long duration of care needs and its provision and does not necessarily designate the place in which the care is being provided.

To get around the heated debates about the meaning of the term, it is sometimes preferable to define the different categories of long-term care:

- Care that can be provided in a community or home setting (so called community-based long-term care) and
- Care that requires a place in which it is provided, with the ultimate and often "classic" concept being a nursing home or comparable setting (often termed institutional or facility-based long-term care).

The problem is, with the growth of the facilities or structures in which such care is provided, it often requires a degree of navigation for a family member and the loved one for whom planning is being undertaken to understand and appreciate the implications of the various components of the long-term care facility-based system. The ethical dimensions related to the issues of long-term care have to do with the decisions required to apply and be accepted and the standards of care expected in the face of ethical principles that govern care. Many people for whom long-term care is necessary or appropriate are not capable to make that decision on their own. They are therefore dependent on surrogates to act on their behalf in the process of applying for and receiving quality care in the context of long-term care, especially when provided in a facility.

I was recently involved in an organization that fits the generally accepted criteria of a "retirement home," some of which in North America provide a range of support services that can accommodate frailer individuals in what is often referred to as an "assisted living" arrangement. The organization was so keen to appear to be different from the formal nursing home (as it is often referred to, especially when part of culturally or religious-based communities) that it did not use the term "retirement home" in advertising. Rather, the promotional material was full of euphemisms about "quality of living" and "respect for individual needs and preferences" such that an unsophisticated reader might not understand the nature of the facility.

What was being advertised appeared to be in contrast to a nursing home, which in some jurisdictions comes under the umbrella of the health care or social service systems. Rather, it was a retirement home with an assisted living section, all of which was privately owned and operated without any financial support or contribution from the government health care delivery systems (managed care and various health maintenance organizations, for example) or public sector.

Whatever setting may be attractive to or suitable for a beloved family member is a matter of individual need, one's financial situation, and sometimes availability, depending on the particular jurisdiction. Urban centers often have many more choices in terms of living options than most small towns or rural settings. In some areas, retirement homes with an assisted living section often provide comparable if not the same services as nursing homes and homes for the aged, as the former may not be available in a way that makes it geographically possible for family members to easily visit their loved ones.

Therefore the reality is that what might be deemed as facilities different from nursing homes may provide comparable ranges of care although under a different funding system—often only privately supported by the families involved in financing the care.

In view of the reality that most formal nursing homes and homes for the aged require some degree of co-payment or in many instances full payment by the clients and patients living in them, the difference in costs may not be as great as expected, but can be substantial. Such details must be clarified before such long-term living arrangements are made by taking into account the financial resources of the person for whom the living arrangement is being made and their family. There is nothing as tragic as having to displace a person from a place where they have become acclimatized in their last period of life and in which they have developed a network and fabric of caring health care professionals and other residents, because of financial considerations.

Because it is a growing industry in response to a greatly expanded population, the issue of quality control and the principles of the contract are important for family members to consider when deciding on a retirement home with or without the assisted living option or a nursing home. The contracts may be different, so it is important to do your homework before making any decisions. A number of independent agencies can be helpful in making choices, and the Internet can be used to find such organizations.

In response to the growing need for and costs involved in long-term care whether in or out of a facility, the long-term care insurance policy has come into being. It can be a useful adjunct in paying the costs of long-term care—but before purchasing be sure that you have compared products and understand the definitions as to what qualifies for coverage.

There are endless stories of individuals who believed the product they purchased would cover the costs in a retirement home only to find by "facility" the insurance policy referred only to nursing homes, for example. Reputable insurance agents and third-party agents can be of assistance in making such decisions. A good review through, for example, the Internet or with the help of a not-for-profit community service or eldercare agency can be most helpful in making such choices and getting reliable information.

Moving into a long-term facility or enhancing community-based long-term care assistance can be an overwhelming decision. It must be considered carefully by all involved in the final decision-making process—include the older individual and all the family members who will be in all likelihood responsible for making sure things work out, whatever decision is made.

Points to Remember

- The long-term care system encompasses community-based and facility-based components. A person may move through different parts of the system at different times of their life.
- The long-term care system is not easy to navigate. Individuals and family members often need help in navigating the system and finding the right combination of facilities and people to fill current and future needs of the person who will need such care.
- Because of the costs of long-term care, whether carried out at home or in a facility, you should explore the various kinds of long-term care insurance to see whether or not it would be worth purchasing. Make sure the contract and what is covered are clear before agreeing to any policy.
- Long-term care arrangements are never easy, even when they are the best that can be achieved. The elder receiving long-term care will continue to require all the support possible from the family to make sure they accommodate to the new living situation.

Who Decides If a Move to a Long-Term Care Facility Is Necessary or Preferred?

The decision to enter a long-term care facility is never easy. Sometimes emotions are deep about such a prospect, especially where there has been some kind of commitment at some time by you and members of your family to respect expressed wishes especially in emotionally charged situations. This may occur, for example, when one older parent is dying and requests to the children, "Please promise that you will never put mother in a nursing home." Or your parent may be very ill and during discussions which might be construed as end-of-life decisions, the subject comes up and the children accede to wishes that are expressed for the future should the illness take a turn for the better. You and your siblings, with emotions running high, usually accede to the request, even though no one can anticipate what might occur in the future and how such a promise might play out in life.

It often happens, whether there was a previous commitment or not, that the situation evolves in such a way that caregiving options change to the point where a long-term care facility might be the only viable alternative for you and your family. To make sure that such a decision is the only possible or reasonable one, it is usually necessary for all the family members to explore their own living situations and recognize what options are available. This may depend on who lives near the older parent. For example, when my father was showing evidence of declining health and function, he lived alone in our family bungalow in Brooklyn, while I lived with my family in Toronto and my sister with hers in Chicago. It was clear that the living situation that would most suit my father's needs would have to be in one of these cities, which my father initially rejected. Later, after important medical events, such a move was accepted as necessary rather than optional.

Separate from the emotional challenges deciding whether a long-term care facility or full-time community-based long-term care is an option, choosing the best arrangement depends on your parent's level of need and the possibilities where they live. The range of possibilities might include living with you or one of your siblings, in their own home with external help and services, living in a retirement home or other assisted living arrangement, or entering a long-term care facility such as a nursing home. In the last case, the degree and intensity of professional health care and medical supervision is the greatest. No one formula fits everyone's needs, but the process should include current and anticipated needs to avoid unnecessary moves from one facility to another. Many organizations have developed programs so that individuals can move within a facility from one level of care to another in the least disruptive and disorientating way.

The first and most critical parts of the process are the discussions that must take place among all of you in the family and the person for whom plans are being formulated. It may not reach resolution the first time around and may be a slow and gradual process. Sometimes it takes a crisis or change in medical condition to propel the decision forward. A serious illness, loss of cognitive function, a broken hip, or a loss of a spouse can be an event that forces decisions to be made more quickly than initially anticipated. Once there is some agreement of the need, the activities necessary to complete the task include getting as much information about the potential facilities available and suitable.

Of the factors that you and your family should consider, one of the most important is the proximity of the facility to those of you who will be involved in ongoing care and visiting. In some areas, especially rural ones, the choices may be limited, but in urban areas there may be many potential choices.

Sometimes help from social agencies that deal with such activities or private individuals who have made careers out of assisting families in such decisions can take the pressure and stress off family members who are struggling with the process. There are also online resources, which have proven to be valuable to those searching for answers. Many provide a wide range of information about facilities and also about challenges related to care provision by families and explore many types of available resources to assist in the process of decision-making and caring.

If and when you and your family members and your parent or parents agree that long-term care is necessary, the process of finding the right place and choosing the right time to move becomes important. An older person's social, ethno-cultural, and sometimes religious affiliations may be of overriding importance in choosing a facility. For that reason, especially in larger urban centers, many choices may reflect the different populations for whom care might be provided.

You and your siblings and other family members have to remember that once a decision is made and a suitable place found, your parent is going to need a lot of support even after moving in. If anything, the involvement of you and your family with the now resident of a long-term care facility is crucial, especially in the early days for proper acclimatization and to establish good and trusting relationships with the care-providing staff.

Points to Remember

- Moving into a long-term care situation is not easy for anyone—not for the older individual or the family.

- Whenever possible, the decision should be a joint one—individual and family.
- Sometimes a crisis in the person's living situation or health needs is required to force the decision to move into a long-term care facility or have full-time help in the community.
- Even after the decision is made for long-term care, family support is crucial to make it a success.

What If the Parent Rejects Help?

Within one day, I had the same conversation with three daughters—one from one family and two from another. "Sometimes you can't plan because the person you are planning for does not want any part of it," was part of my message.

The first was a phone call from the wife of a colleague who had completed a discussion with a health care professional attending to her slightly cognitively impaired mother who was still managing in the community with help. The social worker had said, "There is no planning you (to the daughter) can undertake because your mother is adamant about not leaving her home."

The daughter said to me, "There must be something I can do right now. even if my mother absolutely refuses anything I offer her. She understands up to a point but is so stubborn that I just can't move forward. I am frustrated—I feel I should do something, to plan, but I do not know exactly for what or how."

In the second situation it was two daughters visiting my office with their father who had many medical complaints, all of which were amenable to some beneficial intervention. However, as these were being discussed, including the issue of medication treatment for some depressive symptoms, one of the daughters said, "It is because of the situation at home. My mother is resistant to any assistance from us or anyone else, and this makes things hard for my father. She refuses any help in the house and still expects him, at ninety-two and not as strong as he used to be, to take care of everything."

The daughters acknowledged that they were doing many of the ordinary tasks for their parents, including bill paying and household upkeep. Because their mother refused outside help other than from them, they rotated with another sister and brother who would share in chores rotationally.

"It works, but it is exhausting, and we see the frustration on my father's face every time we try to provide some sort of help and she rejects it. Her memory is poor. Sometimes the same issues come up repeatedly. She refuses to see doctors so that we cannot even find out if some medication might help and she not only fails to take her pills but keeps telling my father he should stop taking his as well."

Such stories are not unusual and for caring children can present an awful ethical and caregiving dilemma—trying to figure out what to do while respecting their parent's wishes, even if they seem irrational. The problem is that even if legally one could remove the decision-making capacity from the parent by nature of mental incapacity, few children are willing to "force" the parent into doing something they vehemently oppose. It is an interesting but important observation that even though many elderly individuals refuse a move to a long-term care facility, in practice many do get moved against what appears to be their wishes and accommodate well and quickly despite their initial opposition.

Sometimes rather than asking your parent to make a permanent choice that will change their living arrangement, it may be acceptable to try something on a temporary basis. Some retirement homes offer a trial period for a few weeks for the person to explore what such a living arrangement is like—a few weeks might not be enough but on occasion a longer trial period might be negotiated.

With my own father, he was reluctant to move from Brooklyn and his own home to a retirement home in Chicago where my sister lived, even though she and I believed it was something that had to be done for his own safety. She arranged a "temporary" stay there for a few months, and he reluctantly agreed to the "trial." While there he had some of his medical problems addressed.

He thought he was well enough to return home to Brooklyn when he was reminded that we had pre-paid for three months. A survivor of the Depression, he wasn't one to throw away money so he agreed to stay until the end of the contract. Fortunately for him and for us, he experienced a medical crisis one night and the ability of my sister to stay overnight with him until it was resolved convinced him to remain there. The morning following the difficult night in question he told my sister, "Sell the house. I am staying here."

Sometimes the children must accept that they cannot force the situation but should keep trying whatever they can think of to cajole, induce, or convince their parent to try something different. At times, the children just have to wait things out until literally "something happens" that causes a crisis that requires intervention. From there things can move forward—the important thing is to recognize that you cannot feel guilty because that is the way it worked out.

One particular case I dealt with involved a physician's parents, both of whom had problems. The father's problems were primarily physical for which a great deal of physical assistance as in dressing and bathing was required. His wife was developing progressive dementia and refused all help in the home and would not even consider moving. The mother fell one day and broke her hip and required hospitalization. A whole cascade of events resulted in the husband being admitted as an urgent respite case to a retirement home for a short term while the wife recovered from her hospitalization.

When it became clear that she required permanent long-term care placement, that was accomplished. The husband joined her at the same multi-level facility but in a different section, so he could visit her. This was not the resolution the daughter had hoped for, but one that occurred while she did the best she could.

As for the daughter noted at the beginning of this section who insisted that she "wanted to do something," in the face of her parent's resistance, I suggested she could explore long-term care facilities so that if and when the time comes, she would know what was available and what might be the best move, without having to explore this option under duress. The important thing to remember is that you can do only what can be done. It is the caring that matters, even when the doing does not go exactly as you might want.

Points to Remember

- It is not uncommon for a parent to reject help that is suggested by even the closest, most loving children.
- Even when legally possible, it is not easy to force older people into unwelcome living situations.
- Repeated offers and examples of help sometimes helps change the person's acceptance of what is required.
- Consider a trial period for a novel living arrangement as one of the ways to see if the parent might accept it without making it permanent from the outset.
- On occasion you can only wait for a crisis to occur, which forces a care situation that resolves the problem for the parent and through the necessary care requirements for the children.

Who Decides Where?

The decision about the best place to move depends on many factors. The primary one should be, whenever possible, to respect the wishes of your loved one for whom the move is being arranged. The ethical concept of autonomy, which underpins much of medical practice, should operate within families as well whenever possible. Complete choice is not always possible, depending on many factors, but when there is a choice and your loved one can participate in it, that should be promoted to the best of your family's ability to do so.

Family needs, financial implications, access and ability to visit and participate after the move has taken place are important and should together influence whatever decision is made.

In many jurisdictions, if the person for whom the move is being arranged cannot participate in such a decision, there is a requirement for an assessment of their capacity to make such a decision—often if not always that assessment is made by a physician. Once that inability determination is made, the family can make the decision on behalf of the person for whom they are acting as surrogate (substitute) decision makers.

The fact that you and your family can legally get the right to move your parent or spouse into a long-term care facility does not make the process any easier. If the person objects strenuously to the move, you and your family must still decide if you will undertake the move despite the voiced objections. Despite your right to make the decision, you can decide if you can put up with all the challenges that exist in keeping your loved one at home. These may include some issues of safety, especially if for example wandering is an issue with potential dangers. With increased modern technologies there are more and more devices to decrease such risks such as sensors and GPS and emergency call systems that may decrease the safety concerns that sometimes motivate families to undertake such moves.

Fortunately, for most frail elders especially those with cognitive impairment, the move into a long-term care facility may be less difficult, challenging, and traumatic than expected. If enough effort and care and visiting are provided by you and your family, especially during the transitional period surrounding the move, and if the facility is supportive of their new resident, most individuals accommodate to their new living situation.

It is important that you and your family are supportive of the move while being firm that moving out is not an option. The use of psychoactive drugs to make the move appear "easier" should be avoided if at all possible as these drugs have significant adverse reactions in many of those who receive them. Rarely, under situations where a move is associated with extreme agitation, medication for short periods might be considered as long as the use is carefully monitored and discontinued after the period of severe behavioral disturbance resolves.

At the end, a move to a well-organized and humanely staffed and caring long-term care facility can add life to years of its elderly clientele rather than the opposite. This is the concern most often expressed by loving family members when faced with the challenge of undertaking such a move against the perceived wishes of the person they love and care for.

Points to Remember

1. Even under the best circumstances a move to a long-term care facility can be a challenging event for all concerned.
2. Depending on the capacity for decision-making of the older person, they may or may not be able to significantly participate in the decision to move or to choose the facility.
3. Getting as much participation as possible from the older person and providing ongoing support after the move are critical to its success.

What Are the Limits to Care?

Families of loved ones admitted to long-term care facilities face many challenges. One of the greatest is what limits if any will be placed on care requested should illnesses or medical crises occur. The flip side of that equation is for facility operators and health care professionals to decide the limits to what care might be offered within the facility.

The questions that occur most frequently usually revolve around whether there should be limits to requests or inclinations by family members to send their loved ones to general hospitals when medical crises occur. These two sides of the equation should be understood clearly as part of the decision to make the move into a long-term care facility. In all likelihood over time issues will arise that will test the basis for such care and highlight the decision-making challenges.

From the perspective of the resident/patient of a long-term care facility, hopefully some discussions, if not written documentation, may have been developed before moving into the facility. If done, you and your family may have a reasonable notion about any limits to care that may be preferred by your loved one on whose behalf you may be acting as a surrogate. The need for surrogate decision-making is most often due to underlying cognitive impairment, dementia, or other brain disorders affecting a loved one—a common phenomenon in many long-term care facilities.

If this dementia exists and some care decisions have been discussed before your loved one moved into a facility, it is usually worthwhile to have discussions with the health care professional staff outlining the range of preferences of your loved one as part of general background. When it comes to urgent medical matters, it is often prudent and desirable to discuss the situation at the time of the event because decisions often do change depending on the exact circumstances of the medical condition.

For example, an opposition in general to acute medical interventions might be modified in the face of a hip fracture, where comfort and pain relief may be the result of surgery rather than improving mobility in a person already using a wheelchair. A bowel blockage may be relieved surgically, not for cure but to avoid an uncomfortable bowel obstruction. Or, in contrast, it may be decided in both of these circumstances to refuse surgery and provide symptomatic pain and other supportive treatment only.

In these circumstances the expectation would be that a comfortable death in a palliative care mode might be preferred to surgical intervention and the possible negative outcomes that often occur and might not be prevented even by technically excellent surgery.

Sometimes it is clear from a person's life-long value system and expressed wishes that under well-defined circumstances health care interventions should be limited to comfort care only, often referred to as palliative care. This is sometimes the case, even when the condition for which it is recommended is not related to a malignant disease, which is the usual cause of a palliative approach especially in the final stages of cancer.

It is reasonable to undertake a palliative approach to care that focuses on symptom management and attention to psycho-social and family needs as part of the roles of those providing professional health care. This approach can be rewarding to those providing the care as well as for those who have requested or accepted the recommendations for such care when the end of life is closing in. This can be so when even the most sophisticated medical technology has little to offer in terms of prolonged life or enhanced function or comfort.

Under such circumstances, families should try to accept the limits of medical interventions and accept the end-of-life period as an important one in terms of providing love, affection, and comfort to those who deserve and require such care. Being able to say after death to your family members and friends that you know that what you did "was right" because you helped provide comfort and support during the final days is an important experience. It is one that will be remembered throughout your lifetime and years after the event.

For health care professionals working in the long-term care setting, there may be a gap between what they feel are reasonable limits to care and what family members often request or at times demand. It is important for health care professionals to understand the reasons for and the values and belief systems that may compel family members to undertake avenues of care that members of the health care staff feel will not provide the outcomes sought by family members. It is important that discussions take place in an atmosphere of support, exploration, and methods to help members of staff understand why decisions that may not make "medical sense" are being taken, and then when possible to provide understanding to family members in the decision-making process.

Sometimes the situation may become adversarial when staff and families do not agree on potential treatments and their implications. Under such circumstances assistance from an organization's ethicist or ethics committee can sometimes help resolve contentious issues. All that can be done to assure that for the last period of life channels of communication and mutual respect and understanding are kept open. Taking whatever steps are necessary to bridge the values gap or expectations gap should be addressed in an open and supportive manner by the health care staff and family members. Sometimes external assistance is required to achieve these ends—it is not always an easy process.

Points to Remember

- All long-term care facilities have limits to the nature of care that they can provide onsite.
- It is important for family members to have a good understanding of what can be provided in the long-term care facility and what would require transfer elsewhere for acute treatment.
- Depending on the nature of the illnesses that might occur for which external transfer might be required, it is useful for family members to have an idea of the limits to which they would want a transfer based on an understanding of the limits to care desired by their loved one.
- When there is conflict between what family members are asking for and what a long-term care facility and its staff in good conscience feel is appropriate in terms of achieving realistic care goals, external assistance from an ethicist or ethics committee might be worthwhile.

15

End-of-Life Care Decisions

Probably nothing is as dramatic or poignant for a family than confronting the reality of a loved one's life ending—even in the face of advanced age, longstanding illness, or dementia. Even when death is expected and at times seems more desirable than a suffering life, the period of life's end is not easy for any family member, no matter how apparently prepared he or she may be.

We often hear people comment when an elderly person dies, "After all, he was eighty-nine and had a good life. What is there to be sad about?" The reality is that children always experience the loss of a parent, however old and however full the life they may have been, as a loss, the end of an era never to be regained. Of course, over time the effect of the loss is usually muted, and most people are good at retaining the positive attributes of the lost parent or other loved one.

In general, what remains are the stories that we incorporate into the fabric of our own lives, with opportunities to remember that person, through various cultural and religious or secular rituals. We often find ways to pass down the legacy of that beloved person to our children and grandchildren through the practice of naming them in their honor or commenting on the similarities in looks or positive or endearing attributes.

All cultures and religions have rituals and practices that help in the end-of-life process. Over the years I have participated in many of them as part of my family and as part of my profession as a geriatrician—although I cannot attend every service after the death of a patient or acquaintance, I have over the years attended many from many religious and cultural backgrounds. The one principle that seems to characterize all of them while in the face of loss is the celebration of the person's life.

I can recall the shock at the first gathering after the burial of my maternal grandmother, which was done at a time when it was not considered "right" to have twelve-year-olds attend funerals or cemeteries. She was dear to me and had helped raise me in a cramped one-bedroom apartment in Brighton Beach shared by her, my sister, myself, and my parents. As family members from all over the country came back to my home after the funeral, I was not surprised with my mother's crying but was astounded that rather than experiencing only gloom I heard peals of laughter. As I listened in to the conversations, I heard snatches of wonderful stories about her that brought joy to everyone that knew her.

The process of end-of-life preparation and decision-making is rarely easy. Each person and family tries to prepare for it in their own way. In some cultures, it is virtually taboo to discuss serious illness or impending death with the person involved as if it would be interpreted as a bad omen and undermines the reverence for that person. In other cultures it is deemed appropriate and even necessary to have open and honest discussions with the person for whom end-of-life decisions are being made and be included in any decisions or plans.

This process depends much on the individuals involved, their patterns of communication, and the comfort with which family members are willing to face the realities of the future. It is important for health care professionals to understand the cultural norms of the families they are dealing with as sometimes conflicts occur when the health care professional believes one type of communication is required when it is not part of the cultural norm for the person involved in the end-of-life decision-making process.

Sometimes it is the formal planning of the end-of-life options and procedures that allows individuals facing their own death along with their loved ones to get through the process. It is not uncommon, for example, on palliative care units for patients to ask health care professionals or palliative care volunteers or clergy to engage with their family members to make sure that everything surrounding the end-of-life period will be taken care of. Many individuals for example plan their funerals in advance to avert the need by their loved ones to make such decisions in the face of great sadness and loss. It can be emotionally trying for a family to decide on the funeral process and type of coffin just after a heart-wrenching death. Because of my professional involvement and recommendations, I have often made such recommendations to other individuals and family members.

In anticipation of my own eventual death, I opted to prearrange my funeral with one of the two major funeral homes in my community. This would mean that my family has only to call the designated number, give my name, and everything will be taken care of. Not only does it give me comfort to know that my family does not have to worry about such details at a time of loss, but also, like most funeral homes that have such programs, the cost is prepaid, which protects my family from any financial considerations, which can be stressful at a time of loss and mourning.

The key to end-of-life decision-making is to communicate as openly as possible about wishes and feelings so that family members and other loved ones can look back and say in one form or another, "We did the right thing. Her death was as good as anyone could hope for. We managed to make her as comfortable as possible. We fulfilled her wishes and values to the best of our ability. We will always remember her for her wonderful qualities, and she will always live in our hearts and memories."

Points to Remember

- End-of-life decisions and the end-of-life period present major challenges to families.
- Communication before the end-of-life period can be helpful when difficult decisions have to be made.
- In some cultures, such discussions would never take place, so family members have to rely on their understanding of their loved one and their own culture and values.
- With the many technologies available, the end-of-life period can be drawn out. Families must do their best to make decisions that are consistent with the values and wishes of their beloved parent so that, after it is over, they can feel that the care provided was the best possible under the circumstances.

Living Wills: Not Always the Answer

Harold, a fifty-two-year-old physician, is the spokesperson for his family, struggling with decisions about Moshe, his eighty-eight-year-old father. Moshe has a long-standing malignant blood disorder, which is in the phase of serious progression. Moshe lives in a long-term care facility. He has been getting some treatment for his blood disorder over the years with the assistance of a hematologist at one of the local general hospitals.

Moshe's physician at the long-term care facility believes that palliative care with comfort measures only is now appropriate because Moshe is gradually declining and the hematologist has told him that there is nothing more to offer in terms of beneficial chemotherapy. The occasional blood transfusions that he had been getting are no longer achieving their goals, even for short periods. Harold feels that further blood transfusions beyond the six he received in the past two months should continue. Harold's three siblings appear to go along, perhaps reluctantly, with him. Moshe's wife, Rivka, says she only wants "the best" for her husband, but as might be expected, defers to her physician son.

During the Schiavo case in the United States, many believed that if there had been a living will (often called an advance directive), the conflict that existed between the patient's husband and his wife's family could have been avoided. But there were no directions.

Moshe, on the other hand, wrote a living will. It contained a lot of detail. It is the interpretation of what Moshe intended when he used the words *comfort measures* and *no heroic measures,* or *being allowed to die peacefully* that is causing conflicts of opinion among Harold and Moshe's physician and the other members of the health care team. They have come to know Moshe over the three years that he has lived with them and been under their care. During this time he had a stroke on top of some degree of dementia that left him at this time incapable of communicating effectively.

Moshe's physician believes that the living will that was written before his moving into the long-term care facility and before he had his stroke indicates a focus on pain and other symptom management. Harold believes that blood transfusions although not curative provide comfort and wants them continued for as long as necessary, while recognizing that they will not alter the course of his father's terminal condition.

He has said, "My father's well-being is what matters most to me, and a blood transfusion is not heroic and provides comfort to him when he gets short of breath because of his anemia." Moshe's physician feels that when shortness of breath becomes a problem, it should be treated in a palliative fashion with medications to address his symptoms and not blood transfusions. He and Harold are at loggerheads.

Here is the situation: a caring and loving family and a dedicated physician are in conflict over the meaning of a written living will. Rather than helping the family and the physician agree on a course of action, the document is causing as much trouble as if nothing at all had been written. Without the document, the same questions about his care might have occurred, but no one would be trying to interpret Moshe's written word to determine treatment.

It would have helped had Moshe explained his intent to his family or to those physicians involved in his care at the time he wrote his living will. He is very sick now and his dementia interferes with his ability to indicate his treatment preferences. Rivka, his wife, who is the legal surrogate and feels that Moshe probably meant that he should be left to die comfortably, has a difficult time disagreeing with her son. This is not just because he is a physician but because she is aware of the close relationship he had with his father and the fervor and determination with which he is making his case—she has found it difficult to express her view to him without him becoming upset and impatient with her and almost accusing her of promoting her husband's premature death.

The last thing any caring family wants in end-of-life situations is conflict, especially if bad feelings after death might be the result. For the treating physician, the true wishes of the patient are usually paramount. When the patient cannot indicate them, physicians must rely on surrogate decision makers who are usually family members. When a living will exists, it is hoped that it will ease the treatment decisions for families and the physician—but as this case indicates, it does not always happen.

There has developed over the past few years an increased belief that living wills (advance directives) may not achieve the goals that they were meant to address. In a July 3, 2007, article published in the prestigious *Annals of Internal Medicine*, "Controlling Death: The False Promise of Advance Directives," well-known scholar Henry S. Perkins concludes, "After thirty years of experience of living wills ... they have not fulfilled their initial promise, which was to remove the uncertainty from end-of-life decisions, avoid family conflicts, and allow individuals to confidently plan their future."

The author postulates the possible reasons such as few people do them in a meaningful and helpful way; there is often ambiguity in the language; the content is often not discussed with those who will have to act on the instructions; and what happens in the world of clinical medicine and end-of-life care cannot be adequately captured in a static document, which cannot have nuance and subtlety which is often the actuality of the situations the documents are supposed to address. At best the documents can be used as support for some thoughts, ideas, and values that family members should try to incorporate in as respectful a manner as possible into the complexity of the decisions that they often have to make for loved ones for whom death is approaching.

The resolution of such a conflict-ridden situation is not always easy. A family meeting with the doctor, a social worker, and maybe an ethicist might help everyone understand the goal of treatment, which is to make Moshe's last days or weeks as comfortable as possible. Respect for his wishes is an important value for the family, so even if he had not explained in detail to anyone why he wrote what he wrote, it appears that he did not want to suffer. As he indicated in the document, he had a good life and wanted a peaceful end. With that in mind, it was possible after lots of soul searching and self-reflection for the family and physician to agree to the limits of future blood transfusions and focus on other comfort measures.

With that approach, Moshe's last days were comfortable, and the family could agree to support each other along with the help of the physician and other health care professional staff during these important final days of what had been a remarkable life.

Points to Remember

- Living wills (advance directives) may have a role in end-of-life planning for decisions about possible treatments.
- If they are of any value, the most important step that has to be taken beyond writing it is to discuss the content and its meaning with family members who are likely going to be interpreting its meaning to the health care professional staff.
- If a living will is to be created, do it with the assistance of your physician(s) to make sure you understand the implications of any phrases that you use such as *heroic* so that your family and those treating you understand what you mean by limits to care and types of clinical interventions.
- Sometimes even in the presence of a living will, there is a conflict in deciding on end-of-life decisions. Meetings with members of the health care professional staff and when suitable the ethics committee or ethicist may make the ultimate interpretation of the living will and the current clinical situation more congruent when final decisions are being made.
- In extreme situations of conflict and disagreement about the meaning and interpretation of living wills, the need for legal adjudication becomes necessary, which usually leads ultimately to a degree of mistrust among the parties. This is unfortunate, as usually a strong therapeutic relationship filled with mutual trust is necessary for end-of-life decisions to meet everyone's needs and wishes for desirable outcomes.

Stopping Treatment: How and Who Decides?

One of the difficult conundrums you and members of your family might face and share with health care professionals is the challenge of discontinuing what might be perceived as life-maintaining treatment, even in the face of the reality that death is inevitable—it is only a matter of time.

Some treatments appear to be complex and the implications dramatic, as when ventilator support is responsible for maintaining life. In such situations it is often the health care teams that recommend its discontinuation, when all clinical indicators support the reality of likely death, even if postponed for short periods by the use of such technologies.

On a more mundane level, the discontinuation of tube feedings is more common and has within it the uncomfortable specter of stopping a basic intervention for which most people feel a duty to continue. In some religions, the obligation to continue feeding is a powerful force that makes families feel that they must carry on even in the face of ultimate death. These same religions may prohibit the discontinuation of technologies such as respirators other than under carefully defined circumstances. They interpret discontinuation at other times is tantamount to euthanasia.

Many legal and ethics scholars have proposed that there is or should be little ethical or legal difference between not starting a potentially life-maintaining treatment and stopping it. Despite these scholarly conclusions, for many health care professionals and family members struggling with such decisions, it seems to be a much more profound step to discontinue, for example, a tube feeding process than deciding not to undertake it at all. For many, the act of commission appears more profound than the act of omission.

One way around the terrible guilt that often accompanies decisions to discontinue life-maintaining treatments that do not appear to achieve their goal other than on a temporary basis is to decide before initiating such treatment whenever possible the framework by which the treatment will be discontinued. If this is laid out by health care professionals with the concurrence of family members at the time, it can more readily be decided that the proposed intervention has not been successful and should therefore be discontinued.

A good example of such a process is that of giving a therapeutic trial of artificial or tube feeding. The goals outlined should be clear from the start: weight maintenance or gain, improvement in nutritional parameters, improved level of consciousness for someone in coma, or some clear clinical evidence of improvement. If the reason for the artificial feeding has a strong religious basis using the concept of "sanctity of life," this too should be discussed with the religious counselor from whom the family is seeking advice. They should make sure that the circumstances are such that what the family perceives as an obligation has some flexibility and decisional capacity by them so it can be built into the ultimate decision.

After time and deliberation, a decision may have to be made to discontinue what may be perceived as potentially life-maintaining treatments. It may come from the health care staff or from the family—there may be congruence in the decision or conflict. In any event, there should be a process with as much respect and communication as possible to allow the decisions to be made and family members supported, not just in their decision but in their feelings about the situation. Unfortunately, at times there is a breakdown in communication and trust between family members and health care professionals. Sometimes a consultation with the facility's ethicist or ethics committee or religious leaders can assuage strong feelings.

Over the years I have been involved in such difficult deliberations with families. In the recent past I had two such family meetings to assist families struggling with decisions about loved ones in serious end-of-life situations. Although in different hospitals with somewhat different illnesses, the basic circumstances were similar.

The children in both families were struggling with whether or not and if so how to "let go." In one family, the parent was in an intensive care unit and one on a regular medical ward in an acute hospital. The prognosis for each one appeared dismal from the perspective of the medical staff. According to the families, the staff indeed had done everything reasonable to salvage their loved one. But things had not gone well and now the end appeared to be at hand—but not quite.

It turned out that both families were Jewish, but I have dealt with similar situations in the past with members of other religions. "We want to do the *right thing* not just as a family but *Jewishly*," they said. In each family the degree of religious observance was modest, and less so than that of the ill parent, but the children's reverence for Jewish values and traditions was high. They had received some informal input from rabbis. They struggled with whether the recommendations of the rabbis truly reflected the values they shared as a family including that of their more traditionally observant parent.

It was not an easy challenge for devoted and loving families. There was a degree of discord between the children. Not all of them were geographically close during the previous number of years, and some did not have the intimate knowledge of their parent as did some of the other more local siblings. Here they were altogether trying to make a decision that they could live with for the rest of their lives.

The question for me was what I might offer in my role as geriatrician and someone who had done post-graduate studies in ethics. I understood the limitations of my formal religious background and training but was also aware of the many situations I had witnessed and my great interest in and respect for the teachings and values within Judaism. I knew that not being a rabbi, my views were a secularized composite and understanding of the cases I had observed and the education I had been involved with over many years of practice. The challenge was mainly at the human level—the struggling with the notion of "letting go" of a beloved member of the family.

How a family deals with such heart-wrenching dilemmas can be addressed from many perspectives—the ethical, the legal, and the personal/family one. Ethically most families want to do the "right" thing. Their understanding of the ethical approach to such decisions is usually a reflection of the principles and values on which they were raised. If they are Jewish or Catholic (or other strongly religious Christian denomination) or Muslim, one often hears that the family wants to respect the religious values of their loved one at the same time as not wanting any avoidable suffering during this end-of-life period. Such concerns are fairly universal across all religions and ethnic groups. Families often struggle with concepts of duties to provide food and drink, often translated into the more clinical "nutrition and hydration," but the association with the loving act of feeding cannot be disregarded. Promoting sanctity of life, a common theme in the three monotheistic religions, often competes with the secular concept of quality of life and avoidance of suffering.

Ontario law as an example of similar laws in North American jurisdictions expects family decisions to reflect what they believe their loved one would have truly wanted or what would be in their loved one's difficult-to-define "best interests." Many family members do not truly know their loved one's wishes and values as such issues are not usually discussed. But it is at the human level that the challenge exists. Time is needed to discuss and explore feelings and values.

At some point it becomes necessary to make a difficult decision. I often counsel families that whatever decision they make is the "right one," whatever the outcome. Second-guessing afterward with "what ifs" is a terrible process that can lead to life-long doubts and recriminations. Talk and feel and share as a family, and then make the best decision that you can. That is all any loving family can do.

In unusual and contentious cases, the situation might require legal intervention, as occurred in the Schiavo case and in the well-known cases that went to the U.S. Supreme Court (*Cruzan* and *Quinlan*). Fortunately, such cases are unusual. Most family and health care providers share sufficient mutual respect and caring for the results to be acceptable so that, after the fact and years later, family members can live with and look back on a profound and ethically and emotionally charged experience. Hopefully it would have been one from which they learned and matured in their understanding of life and illness and of their own values, vulnerabilities, and strengths.

Points to Remember

- Stopping treatment, especially what is interpreted to be life-saving or life-maintaining, is never easy for families.
- Modern medicine has many technological interventions that can maintain people's lives even when it is most unlikely that any meaningful long-term recovery would take place.

- Even when it is understood by the family that death is likely to occur, the agreement to discontinue such therapy can cause enormous emotional conflict.
- Sometimes cultural or religious values make it even more difficult to discontinue such life-saving or life-maintaining treatments, even in the face of likely long-term failure of effectiveness of such treatment.
- Communication among family members and health care professionals with at times external assistance and support may be required to ultimately come to final decisions. It is hoped that, in meeting the goals and values of the caring family, decisions can be made without compromising important ethical principles in the provision of care such as the avoidance of prolonged suffering.

16

Palliative Care: Achieving the Goals of Comfort and Dignity

End-of-life decisions are always difficult for patients and families and may result in conflicts. Even when the goals of treatment have apparently been agreed to and palliative care is decided upon, problems may occur. In such circumstances, it might seem easy to decide on end-of-life pain and other symptom management, but at times difficulties arise in the achievement of these domains of care, which require understanding and communication with patients and family members as well as a strong element of trust.

One particular case was of special interest as an example of the different perspectives that often come together when there are misunderstandings and discordance in goals of palliative and end-of-life care and when the personal and professional perspectives may not be immediately congruent.

The daughter asked to speak to me about her mother, who was in a nursing home. The family had expressed a desire on her behalf that she be able to stay there if possible until her death, rather than be transferred to another facility, even one connected to the nursing home. The daughter was concerned because she felt that even though there had been a good ongoing relationship with her mother's attending physician for a number of years, the recent change in her mother's care needs and the family's requests had led to a degree of temporary conflict with him.

The resolution finally did take place. But the daughter felt that the issue in general had to be addressed so that in the future there would be a smoother and more receptive response to palliative care and end-of-life needs rather than the standard investigational and treatment approach that had been the basis of the previous medical issues as it concerned her mother.

Ironically, soon after this particular discussion, at an ethics seminar, the same case was presented from the perspective of young physicians undergoing post-graduate training. The family practice resident (in her first of two years of post-graduate training) said she had a difficult case she wanted to bring to the ethics seminar group.

The resident presented her case: "I was involved in a consultation about a resident of the Home for the Aged in which there seemed to be a difference in opinion and focus on the needs for palliative care and pain management as opposed to tests to try to provide further clinical information." As the case unfolded, the group in the ethics seminar acknowledged that issues related to end-of-life care are often the focus of ethical deliberation. This seemed to be the case because they appeared to appreciate that, from their training already, the stress on patients, families, and staff is often greater than might occur in other domains of clinical practice and care.

The medical resident continued, "It seems that the family had strong feelings about the kind of care they believed they should be providing for their mother based on her communications with them before she became extremely ill. They felt at this point, irrespective of the cause of her symptoms, they wanted palliative care and a commitment to pain management, as she appeared to be suffering. They were unhappy that she was receiving minimal pain medication and nothing that had substantial opiate effectiveness."

As the story unfolded, it seemed that the primary care physician was concerned that the cause of the pain was not clear. One of the consultants had recommended some tests, and the doctor was of the opinion that palliative care steps should not be taken until such time that it was clear what was going on.

The geriatric medicine consultant for whom the family practice resident had seen the patient believed that a pain-management evaluation was in order and requested that it be undertaken. The resident continued, "When a recommendation for graded morphine doses was made, that resulted in some reluctance from the attending physician, because of the previous concern."

The question that became the focus of the ethics seminar discussion was this: What is the basis by which end-of-life decisions are made? What does one do if members of the health care staff, whether physicians or nurses, are uncomfortable implementing treatment with opiates because of the fear that it could be misconstrued as causing death and be the basis of professional regulatory or legal action?

This of course is just one perspective of the case, the other being what are the feelings and sensibilities of the family who feel that their parent is not getting necessary pain management and might be experiencing unnecessary suffering.

Among the issues to be addressed in the ethics-based discussion were the role and responsibility of the surrogate in interpreting the wishes of the patient and the role and responsibility of the physician in responding to those wishes as expressed by the family members in their role as surrogates.

Another issue is whether the provision of pain-management medications such as morphine, which might marginally hasten death while providing symptom management, could be interpreted as being a means for unprofessionally and prematurely ending a life and as providing euthanasia, which is illegal in Canada and the United States. (Note: Physician-assisted suicide, which is clearly distinguished from euthanasia, is legal only in Oregon, Washington and Montana under strict criteria.) Could a request by a family member for what might be misconstrued as excessive pain control be misinterpreted as the family wanting the end to occur more quickly than might be clinically necessary or appropriate, given the prohibition of life-ending interventions on the part of physicians?

The first issue has to be addressed within the framework of respect for patient autonomy either directly when possible or through a surrogate when the patient is no longer able to communicate directly. Health care professionals rarely can question the basis by which surrogates express the needs of those for whom they are speaking. The attempt to get individuals to complete advance directives/living wills has not resulted in a huge upsurge in this activity. Even when those wishes are written down, the documents often merely confirm who would be the surrogate and maybe deal with some major interventions, such as tube feeding or CPR.

Thus, family members who make up the majority of surrogates are left with their understanding of the wishes based on their long-standing knowledge of the family member, the underlying values (religious or otherwise), and conversations that they have shared on the subject of end-of-life planning. It is not uncommon for older individuals to tell their children what they would want at the end of their lives and give a reasonable basis for their children to make caring and informed decisions about end-of-life care. Even when some instructions are given, they rarely address details of treatments but rather focus understandably on broad goals of care.

I usually recommend to family members to have those important and frank conversations with their parents about what their wishes might be if conditions result in serious illness for which little hope of recovery exists or, even with recovery, if function will be severely compromised.

Sometimes it is hard for the parent to express wishes and details. In such circumstances, I have found it useful to explain to the parent what the children believe he or she would want under given circumstances. I recommend framing the conversations something like this, "As (name the siblings) and I have known you for so many years, it is important that we know what you would want if your condition becomes so severe that there is little hope for return to full or normal function. (It is useful here to use an example of someone who went through it, such as a friend or relative.) From our understanding of you and your life values and everything you have told us over the years, we believe that if you should be in such a situation, you would like us to withhold or withdraw treatment and let nature take its course and make you comfortable." (Or, if the values are different, for example, for religious reasons, the result might be, "Do everything possible to keep you alive with as little suffering as possible in keeping with your strong religious beliefs.")

From the perspective of the physician, it is always worthwhile when discussing decisions being made by surrogates to ask in as supportive and sensitive way as possible why a decision by a surrogate is being made. In the case noted here, the children were united and adamant that their mother had clearly told them that she did not want any more tests and treatments, that she had lived a full life and wanted to be allowed to die. She also had told them that she had pain and wanted it treated, either directly or through her expressions of suffering from the pain she was currently experiencing.

Although the family understood that the cause of the painful symptoms was not clear and that there might have been some identifiable and treatable conditions that the physician was focusing on, they believed that their mother did not want any further tests. Rather the focus was to be on symptom and pain control so that the last days and hours of her life could be peaceful and free of suffering. Because the mother had some degree of cognitive impairment, the physician was not comfortable accepting her own expression of such wishes to her, which did occur, and preferred to turn to the family members for instructions. Such expressions as the basis of a surrogate's decision-making process should normally have great weight in the physician's direction of care.

The next important issue with which many physicians struggle, especially those who are not experienced in the principles and practices of palliative and terminal care, is how does one administer morphine and other narcotic (opiate) medications in such a way as to meet the symptom control requirements of the patient without appearing to hasten death, especially when larger doses than might be usually given for other types of pain may be required for end-of-life pain management. This becomes even more difficult when the symptoms in question may be less dramatic than pain but be, for example, severe shortness of breath for which narcotics can also be helpful.

Many physicians fear the use of narcotics. The stringent regulations on the use of this class of medication in many jurisdictions, especially in North America, are a reflection of the concern that society, law enforcement agencies, and the regulatory professional groups have on inappropriate use of such drugs. There is also a substantial illegal use of the drugs and concerns in the general population about the addictive properties of the drugs. These two views converge into an inherent ambivalence on their use other than by physicians who have gained comfort in their appropriate use. It is these physicians who are most comfortable with their use and know how to adjust dosages to meet therapeutic end-of-life and pain/symptom-management goals without compromising their professional responsibilities and standards of care or that might put them in regulatory or legal jeopardy.

Gaining the knowledge of pain relievers and their use, including opiate and other symptom-management drug therapies, should be an important goal of all physicians who might become involved in end-of-life and palliative care. It is often a luxury, not always available, to transfer all potential patients who need palliative care to special units or programs such as dedicated hospice units that like palliative care programs exist in many jurisdictions. Therefore, for many primary care physicians, the challenges and professional responsibility fall on them.

In addition to the knowledge and comfort level in the use of narcotic medications directed to palliative and terminal care pain management, regulatory bodies understand that at times large doses of narcotics might be necessary to adequately control terminal-disease-related symptoms. In general, what the regulatory bodies look for in their quest to make sure that physicians are fulfilling their ethical, professional, and legally based roles is to understand the basis and grounds by which the narcotic dosage was achieved, rather than the specific dose provided at any given time.

For example, providing a patient with subcutaneous morphine at the dose of 30 mg every four hours with 10 mg every two hours for breakthrough pain, which resulted in death two days after the dose was written, would likely be considered appropriate care rather than the institution of euthanasia. If such a case came to an inquiry, it would be the basis of the dosing and the fact that it was incrementally increased with documented results of the preceding doses in terms of adequacy of pain management that would be the measure.

The concept that death may be hastened by the provision of appropriate narcotic palliative pain management has long been accepted as ethically and legally sound and probably occurs far less commonly than believed. The crux of the argument is the intent of administering the drug. Giving a patient with palliative care needs, who had not previously been exposed to narcotics for pain management, a large dose that clearly resulted in a rapid demise would probably be looked on with suspicion, especially if there was inadequate documentation as to the goals of therapy and the process by which the goals were to be achieved.

An article published in the December 2006 issue of the *Journal of Pain and Symptom Management* from the National Hospice and Palliative Care Organization has challenged and appears to have dispelled the belief that the administration of opiates (including morphine) hastens death under the usual circumstances of its use in this palliative/terminal patient population. Because of this erroneous belief, the adequate administration of pain-reducing opiate medications are often denied—this apparently misconstrued belief can be a significant barrier to effective pain management for dying patients.

The study suggests that the timing of death among patients with advanced illness involves a complex interplay of variables and that effective opiate use poses little risk of hastened death. The authors go on to explain that undertreatment of pain is a far more pressing concern than is the risk of hastened death in those with advanced disease. Available research indicates that physicians should be encouraged to use opiates effectively to relieve suffering at the end of life.

The study examined outcomes of seven hundred twenty-five hospice patients who were receiving opiates and had at least one change in dose before death. The study looked at both the total daily amount of opiate given and the changes in dose on the timing of death. Opiate dosing explained little of the variation in survival time among these patients. The study concluded that concern about hastening death does not justify withholding opiate therapy.

Stephen Connor, co-author of the study and a well-known palliative care researcher said, "Most clinicians understand the value of using opiates to relieve suffering at the end of life but fear of hastening the death of seriously ill persons contributes to unnecessary suffering. This study reassures clinicians that their effective use of opiates in the seriously ill will not hasten death and will lead to better quality care. We all want to be kept comfortable and pain free at the end of our lives."

Many patients in need of end-of-life palliative and terminal care pain management do not receive such care. Despite much being written on the subject and initiatives taken to try to rectify the situation, the medical profession has not yet reached the point where we can assure the patient population that they do not need to suffer from pain that could likely be controlled with appropriate pain medication. It is the ethical and professional responsibility of physicians to make sure that they have the knowledge and commitment to make sure that they can respond to the end-of-life pain management needs of our patients.

As a family member, it is important to understand the dynamics and conflicts that may exist in providing appropriate palliative end-of-life care, especially in the domain of pain management. If your loved one happens to have access to a palliative care program, these issues are usually appropriately addressed and necessary treatment is usually provided. If such a unit or program is not available, it may be necessary for you to work with the physicians and other health care professionals to make sure that they understand the basis of your goals and the commitment to make sure that your loved one's last days are free of unnecessary suffering and relieved of treatable symptoms, including pain, whenever possible.

Points to Remember

- Palliative care is a philosophy of care rather than a place—although much of this type of care takes place in palliative care or hospice units. Such care should be able to be provided anywhere in the long-term care system, but this is not always the case.
- The goal of palliative care is to control the pain and other symptoms of patients in the terminal stages of life.
- Once palliative care is agreed to, acute interventions should no longer be considered and would be deemed unsuitable within the context of meeting the end-of-life needs of those whose illnesses are no longer responsive to such interventions.
- It is generally a precondition for a palliative care program that acute care interventions will not be undertaken.
- The goal is to relieve suffering and sometimes the implications of such care are the use of strong pain-relieving medications, which may cloud consciousness as part of the process of achieving comfort.
- If you have a loved one in a palliative care program, discuss with the staff what you might expect from the course of the disease and the type of symptoms and issues that might occur during your loved one's final weeks, days, and hours.

17

Ethical Perspectives of Health Care Professionals

Patients and families struggling with many of the clinical and ethical issues that are likely to occur in the later stages of life may not seem particularly interested in the ethical issues that affect health care professionals. However, to understand and appreciate the process by which health care professionals participate in the care of those you love, it is worthwhile to explore some of the challenges that they experience while trying to fulfill their professional and ethical responsibilities.

For people who do not have personal experience with health care professionals as family members or friends, it may be hard to fathom what goes into being a member of a health care profession. The public has many beliefs about what it means to be a doctor or nurse or social worker or rehabilitation therapist, but little clear understanding of the ethical and professional framework that those in the various fields are expected to heed in their professional practices.

Sometimes even those in the field may be uncertain as to how they are expected to act in certain challenging circumstances of clinical responsibility. The contemporary practices of medicine have introduced so many new options and technologies that it might be a daunting challenge for health care practitioners to be cognizant of all the nuances of ethical and professional practice and the legal frameworks, which are constantly undergoing change as new cases come forward and change the legal and often the political climate in which all health care professionals must work.

An example is the controversy and historical and legal developments about the ability to discontinue life-maintaining treatments. It took a number of U.S. Supreme Court rulings before a family member could request the discontinuation of tube feedings or respirators, so health care professionals were obligated to follow those instructions, assuming that all the necessary criteria for such decision-making were in place. For health care professionals who were trained and spent much of their clinical experience in a structure that disallowed such decisions by family members, it can be a major challenge to shift gears not only in the process of decision-making but in the communication process with family members.

Over the years, all of the health care professions have developed ethical frameworks of practice and what are often referred to as Codes of Conduct. These outline for each member what can be expected by the general community and other health care colleagues when it comes to decision-making and care provision of patients. An example is the so-called "best interests" principle by which health care providers should understand and use when there might be a conflict within the decision-making paradigm—the patient for whom actions are being taken must always be considered central to the decision-making process.

For those working in health care structures in which there might be financial and other resource utilization demands on the health care providers, it is easy to understand the dilemmas and challenges often faced by health care professionals beyond the more common real or potential disagreements between themselves and family members when some difficult end-of-life decisions have to be contemplated.

Ultimately it is important for the public to appreciate and recognize that the overwhelming majority of those individuals who enter the health care professions do so out of a desire to be helpful to those they will serve. They act out of the ethical sense and principle of beneficence (supporting the "good" in patient care), which is a powerful motivating force for those who choose to be health care professionals.

In addition to their own motivations to act out of professional and ethical duties and obligations, most jurisdictions have developed fairly sophisticated measures and processes and policies to help health care professionals follow their natural motivations and internalized principles of being part of a "caring" profession. Most family members would likely concur that those that they have entrusted with the well-being of a loved one have taken on the responsibility in an ethically respectful and professionally admirable fashion.

Points to Remember

- It is important to try to understand the perspective and challenges of health care professionals in order to understand what drives them to provide the best care possible for your loved one.
- Health care professionals have many demands made on them while trying to fulfill their caregiving role.

- By understanding the various issues that health care providers must contend with, family members can better communicate with them in ways to maximize their ability to care for their parents who are after all the professionals' patients.

The Duty of Health Care Professionals to Be Vaccinated

An example of the duties and obligations of health care professionals that fall into an ethical framework is the concept of the duty to be vaccinated against potentially communicable diseases. There is a long history and debate among the public as to the necessity and duties of ordinary citizens to be vaccinated and for parents to have their children vaccinated. But that issue is not the focus of the current concern. It is whether for health care professionals the duty for their own vaccination is something that should be of ethical and professional concern to the public. The public at special risk includes elders and their families who come into contact with these same health care professionals when they are with their elderly family members.

One might think that the benefits compared to the risks of vaccination appear to justify professionally, ethically, and from the perspective of public health a requirement that all health care providers be vaccinated against the common communicable disease such as the yearly influenza strains. However, that is not always the case. It is not always easy to sort out what must be done to assure that health care providers follow through on what many feel is part of their professional duties.

It was months before the 2003 SARS outbreak in Ontario. The posters about getting the "flu shot" were being posted. I casually reminded a nurse, whom I had known for a number of years, to be vaccinated.

"I never get the vaccine," was her response.

"Why not?" I asked, surprised, because there was so much hype about the vaccination program, especially in hospitals and long-term care facilities.

"I never get the flu and I don't like injections," she said.

Puzzled and disappointed, I discussed her stance with a number of her colleagues who confirmed it was not uncommon among nurses and other health care staff. I had previously made a presentation on influenza vaccinations at an ethics workshop for infection control health care providers, including nurses. Those present recognized that low vaccination rates among some health care provider populations was a major challenge—one for which no one had a good solution.

In recent years, a paramedic in Ontario challenged the provincial requirement that emergency medical service staff be vaccinated. Even though many in the field felt it was important to pursue the case legally, it was eventually dropped. As a result, there are currently no standards or regulatory systems to mandate health care professionals to receive a yearly influenza vaccination in the province of Ontario. That same situation exists in most jurisdictions in the United States.

This presents clinical and ethical challenges to the long-term care system and to all health care professionals, especially given the potential for further SARS outbreaks like the one that hit Toronto, which caused havoc among everyone living in the city at the time, especially among the health care professionals who were put at risk on a daily basis. The concern in 2009 about the H1N1 (swine flu) epidemic raised the same types of concerns.

For the frail elderly populations in long-term care facilities, influenza can cause serious illness or death. It is common for many facilities to get an almost 100 percent vaccination rate among the residents and patients, which should provide substantial protection against influenza. However, because of compromised immune systems, either due to age or illness, the response to vaccination is less robust in the frail elderly than in younger people. Therefore, despite excellent client vaccination rates, outbreaks still occur in long-term care facilities with resultant serious illness and death.

Clinically, there is no longer any question that the vaccination of health care staff, especially those who go from patient to patient, is one of the key steps for prevention of seasonal influenza outbreaks, especially among vulnerable populations. Vaccinating the staff is key to decreasing the risk of infection to individual clients and to preventing outbreaks that can move through a unit with such force that many patients and residents succumb to a largely preventable infection.

Because the initial symptoms of influenza, both seasonal and H1N1 and SARS are indistinguishable, we should be doing everything possible to decrease the incidence of influenza, if only so we don't find ourselves closing down health care facilities and introducing large-scale quarantines because we are not sure of the diagnosis. By having fewer cases of influenza, we are decreasing the likelihood of considering an outbreak to be SARS when it might be influenza.

From the professional and ethical perspective, one would expect health care professionals to understand that they have duties and obligations to themselves and to their patients that would result in their being vaccinated (except, of course, under rare circumstances when a true allergy to such vaccines has been demonstrated). It could be expected that when the vaccination was made available, all staff would come forward to participate, based on their knowledge of what is required to protect patients and residents. But this has not been the case for many years even when excellent programs exist to make the vaccination readily available to all health care professionals at no financial cost to themselves.

The real question is whether a staff member who does not agree to be vaccinated despite their understanding of the clinical information has any professional and ethical basis to comply with vaccination as part of their professional role. If they do not comply, what steps are reasonable to take? How do we make sure the health care professional staff is vaccinated without having to go through weeks of requesting, cajoling, begging, enticing, and bribing with gifts and prizes? (These are all methods that have been used over the past few years in various health care and long-term care facilities to get staff to agree to vaccination.)

What if being vaccinated, because of its important public health impact and because it protects the people we care for, were a requirement and a condition for work? Does that in any way unduly compromise the individuality and personal choice of the health care provider?

Within the realm of public health, we generally agree that the good of the community or society exceeds that of the individual. For example, reporting requirements exist for illnesses that otherwise would not be communicated to a third party. And we put immunization requirements on children's eligibility to enter public schools to protect the community of students and staff.

Although cases of influenza may occur despite large-scale immunization, the benefits appear to justify professionally, ethically, and from the perspective of public health, a requirement that all health care providers be immunized against influenza as a condition for working in the system. Influenza vaccinations have become of increased importance after the outbreaks of SARS and are likely to increase in importance because of the H1N1 strain. Given the horrendous potential impact on patient care, the economy, and the whole health care community, can we in the health care professions ethically refuse?

There are some scholars, a number from the United States, who believe that it would be wrong and ineffectual to make vaccination mandatory for health care staff. They have cited issues of autonomy as well as concerns about alienating staff whose numbers are few in the system. They have also cited concerns about legal liability should a health care worker become ill after receiving a vaccination. Although such arguments might seem compelling, they appear minor when compared to the negative effect of an influenza outbreak, which could be promoted by an unvaccinated health care provider.

Points to Remember

1. Vaccination of health care staff is an important example of looking at practices and policies that affect professionals who provide care to our elderly loved ones through the lens of ethics and professional duties.
2. Good evidence supports the observation that the higher the vaccination rates are among the health care staff who care for elders in long-term care, the lower the infection rate among those who live in long-term care facilities.
3. Getting health care professionals to voluntarily agree to vaccination has not been as successful as once hoped for. Not all see their professional duties in such a way to sacrifice their own autonomy to be vaccinated and thereby protect those they care for.
4. There are arguments for and against the concept of mandatory vaccination for health care staff. The idea is to assure that the frail elders they look after who are most vulnerable to communicable infections—influenza, for example—are maximally protected by having the health care staff that provides care vaccinated on a yearly basis. Many feel that should be part of public policy.

Conflicts with Patients and Families

In many ways, much of what has been addressed in previous sections of this book has a direct or indirect goal of decreasing the risk of major and insurmountable conflicts between patients and families. It is understandable in emotionally charged situations where the well-being of your loved one is at stake that family members may find issues of concern. They enter into the relationship with health care professionals responsible for providing necessary and at times what is perceived to be life-maintaining care in a state of heightened suspicion or doubt as to whether adequate care is being provided.

There are many reasons to explain how this might happen. One of the core features is a lack of adequate communication between families and health care staff as to expectations and values. With the pressure of work and often understaffed units, the time required for personal exploration is often limited. There is also the issue of the kind of appreciation and respect that most family members believe is appropriate to receive from health care professionals for whom most individuals hold with a great deal of de facto respect for their professional status, knowledge, and experience. When a health care professional acts in a condescending or apparently off-handed way, or there are different explanations for the same events, family members can lose confidence in the health care team, or in some members of the team.

Conflicts between families and health care professionals can undermine the goals of treatment and care. Although they often occur, sometimes at profound and at other times relatively minor levels, anything that compromises the trust that family members want to have in those caring for the loved ones is counterproductive. Such suspicion of lack of dedication, knowledge, or trust when held by family members can make even the most basic health care decisions contentious, often promoting a vicious cycle of mistrust and an adversarial relationship. At the extremes, you may hear words like "complaint to professional regulatory bodies" or "sue" when the situation seems to spiral out of hand.

Most organizations have ways to intervene to reestablish trust between the parties involved. This is often done through an administrative mechanism and increasingly often these days by using ombudspersons, ethicists, and ethics committees to help identify the issues about the source of the mistrust. With the deliberative process, especially when framed around ethical principles that health care professionals and family members can agree to subscribe to, an eventual meeting of the minds and forging of common goals and approaches can be developed.

With such an approach to defusing existent or potential conflicts, the goals of care, which are meeting the needs of the loved one whose care is in question, can usually be achieved. It is most important that health care providers and family members find common ground in respect for what might appear to be disparate goals so that the most important person within the potential or real situation of conflict—the patient (beloved family member)—is not forgotten. It is important to avoid allowing recriminations to become the focus of discussions and deep feelings and subsequent actions. They should not be allowed to replace a mutual caring and supportive approach to patient care.

18

The Final Journey

Many issues challenge the relationship and decision-making processes that involve elders and their families. Illness and expected disability or death is often a cauldron that either brings families together or further causes dissent among the various members. All families have complex relationships that over the years either bring a special cohesiveness or antipathy or, in most cases, a combination of both.

No two families are the same, and no two medical situations are exactly the same, although similar patterns do recur as in most issues affecting individuals and their families. For those involved in caregiving and for those on the receiving end of such care, it is important to remember that we must always try to maintain openness to the individual and their distinctive approach to their lives and their relationships. It is within this expansive context of human relationships that all involved should endeavor to approach the challenges that are offered to us throughout our lives and that are especially highlighted during times of stress in response to illness and more so with impending or possible death.

With time and experience and the maturity that we hope to accrue from life, it is hoped that as we face the complex challenges of watching our parents age and perhaps decline cognitively that we will be able to respond effectively and humanely. As we experience the many losses that may accompany aging, we should become ready to respond in a loving and supportive fashion. Most people, whatever their background, their cultural associations, or religious beliefs, want to do the "right" thing when it comes to assisting their elder loved ones in making critical decisions as they age. The narrative of each person is unique, and how families interface and interact with that person's story is an individual happening.

We all hope that we have the strength, foresight, good fortune, and fortitude to experience those life events in such a way that, when we look back, we can feel satisfied that we fulfilled our mandate and duties as loving family members. We can all hope that those who will care for us will undertake their own responsibilities in a similar manner.

Glossary of Commonly Used Ethical Terms

Advance care planning: Includes making decisions about the type of personal care, including health care, living arrangements, food, clothing, hygiene, and safety, that you want to receive in the future. This can be done by preparing a Power of Attorney for Personal Care or Health Care Power of Attorney (term commonly used in the United States) in which you name a substitute decision maker and provide whatever information is believed to be pertinent to future decision-making.

Advance directive or living will: A written document in which you clearly specify treatment preferences and how medical decisions affecting you are to be made if you are unable to make them. It usually also authorizes a specific person (surrogate decision maker) to make such decisions on your behalf when you are no longer able to make such decisions because of mental incapacity.

Artificial nutrition and hydration: A form of life-sustaining treatment. It is a chemically balanced mix of nutrients and fluids provided by placing a tube directly into the stomach, the intestine, or a vein.

Autonomy: One of the foundational ethical principles. It says that each person should be involved in making personal choices and to have his or her choices respected within the bounds of the law, institutional values and policies, and the sensibilities of staff and other clients. Clients'/patients' wishes should be solicited whenever possible and will be an essential component of health care decision-making or when planning care or following instructions in an advanced directive/living will.

Beneficence: Another foundational principle of medical ethics. Each staff member is obliged to do "good," to promote others' welfare and well-being, in accordance with the health care professionals' code of ethics and professional duties and obligations.

Best interest standard: A judgment based on an idea of what would be most beneficial to a patient, usually pursued in the absence of a patient's expressed wishes.

Cardiopulmonary resuscitation (CPR): An emergency procedure consisting of external cardiac massage and artificial respiration; the first treatment for a person who has collapsed and has no pulse and has stopped breathing—attempts to restore circulation of the blood and prevent death or brain damage due to lack of oxygen.

Codes of conduct/ethics: see Professional code of ethics.

Competent (also referred to as capable): A legal concept that describes people who are able to make their own decisions. Minors are presumed to be incompetent, except under certain specified conditions. The corollary medical-ethical term is *decisional capacity*.

Distributive justice: One of the foundational ethical principles. It is concerned with the fair allocation of resources among all members of a target community. Fair allocation generally includes the total amount of goods to be distributed, the distributing procedure, the conceptual support for the procedure, and the pattern of distribution that results.

Duty: The special responsibility associated with a particular profession or occupation or societal role. Physicians, journalists, students, or parents all have special duties. The duty of an individual or group includes descriptions about how the duty makes the group different from other groups in the society. This is also a key term in Kantian ethics: We have a duty to abide by the moral law built into our minds. Compromises and little white lies are not permissible.

Ethical dilemma: A moral conflict that involves determining appropriate conduct when an individual faces conflicting professional values and responsibilities.

Ethicist: One whose judgment on ethics and ethical codes has come to be trusted by some community, and (importantly) is expressed in some way that makes it possible for others to mimic or approximate that judgment. Professionals who are skilled in helping people make decisions about what is morally right and wrong.

Ethics committee: An interdisciplinary group that deals with conflicts of values in patient care in acute and long-term settings. Such committees discuss policy issues (for example, regarding withholding and withdrawing of life-sustaining treatments).

Euthanasia: The act of either permitting a person to die or intentionally ending a person's life generally rooted in motives of mercy, beneficence, or respect for patient dignity.

Informed consent: The legal and ethical requirement that no significant medical procedure can be performed until the competent patient has been informed of the nature of the procedure, risks and alternatives, as well as the prognosis if the procedure is not done. The patient must freely and voluntarily agree to have the procedure done.

Justice: Each person has a right to be treated fairly, in the process of making decisions (procedural justice) or in the way limited resources are allocated (distributive justice). Procedural justice is reflected when all interested parties have an opportunity to be heard and all options are explored when making decisions. Distributive justice considers access to health care and social service resources based on the various components of need.

Life-sustaining treatments: Used to maintain life in circumstances that without such treatments life is likely to end with the usual understanding that such treatments are often temporary in nature until a person recovers from a serious illness or until a decision is made about future treatments. Examples of life-sustaining treatment include, but are not limited to, mechanical ventilation, renal dialysis, chemotherapy, and the administration of artificial nutrition and hydration.

Nonmaleficence: Another foundational ethical principle. Health care professionals are obliged whenever possible to prevent or do no harm. Nonmaleficence is linked to beneficence when health care professionals are (1) not doing evil nor causing harm, (2) preventing evil or harm, or (3) removing evil or sources of harm and thereby promoting good.

Palliative care: Medical or comfort care that reduces the severity of a disease or slows its progress rather than providing a cure. For incurable diseases, in cases where the cure is not recommended due to other health concerns, and when the patient does not wish to pursue a cure, palliative care becomes the focus of treatment. Among other things palliative care strives to accomplish the following: provide relief from pain and other distressing symptoms; affirm life and regard dying as a normal process; intend neither to hasten or postpone death; integrate the psychological and spiritual aspects of patient care; offer a support system to help patients live as actively as possible until death.

Passive euthanasia: Intentionally allowing a person to die by withholding or withdrawing treatment or by permitting the disease process to progress without further intervention. It is sometimes difficult to differentiate the natural course of disease from an act whose purpose is to specifically and intentionally promote death.

Power of Attorney for Personal Care (term commonly used in Canada), or **Health Care Power of Attorney** (term commonly used in the United States): A document in which you name a person or more than one person to be responsible for making personal decisions on your behalf should you become incapable. The person named on the document is known as the Attorney for Personal Care. You can also provide written instructions about the type of personal care that is preferred or rejected at some point in time in the future should incapacity occur. Decisions about life-sustaining treatments such as ventilators, intensive care, and intravenous and tube feeding may be included.

Principlism: An approach to ethical thinking established in the 1970s that approaches ethical issues through a number of principles that allow a deliberative approach to understanding and resolution. These four foundational principles include respect for autonomy, nonmaleficence, beneficence, and justice.

Professional code of ethics: Professions are powerful social groups that have been assigned the responsibility to use their power for the good of the less powerful. A code of ethics is a formal statement that both claims that responsibility and gives guidance to its accomplishment. A code of ethics guides the responsible action of the professional.

Professional values (or duties): All health care professional groups have identified a set of expectations for each of their members. These expectations are based on what the professional group has agreed are the most important values, or virtues, to be maintained. Integrity, respect, and compassion are commonly cited as virtues expected of health care professionals.

Quality of life: Often contrasted with quantity or sanctity of life and indicates that there are moral limits to the use of life-prolonging medical interventions. Quality of life is regarded as a patient-centered moral criterion, emphasizing the worth of the patient's own life to himself or herself.

Substituted judgment: A process whereby a proxy makes a decision about medical treatment for an incompetent patient based on his or her understanding of what the patient would have decided if competent. The substituted judgment standard has been important in influential legal decisions and is typically contrasted with the *best interest* standard.

Surrogate decision maker: A person or persons who will make decisions on behalf of an incapable person. Persons who are incapable are not able to understand the nature of treatment choices or appreciate the consequences of their decisions.

Ventilator: A breathing machine that is used to treat respiratory failure by promoting ventilation; also called a respirator.

Veracity: Each person is entitled to be told the truth, to the extent he or she wishes to know it. Caregivers expect truthful and accurate information from clients and their families. A relationship based on truth and sharing information in an objective, accurate, and comprehensive manner fosters trust among clients, their families, and health care professionals. This mutual trust is the essential element in relationships formed to meet the common goal of enriching the quality of life of the client and providing the highest quality of care.

Vulnerable patient (or person): Vulnerable means wounded and unable to defend oneself. Patients have a strong self-perception of vulnerability, but truly vulnerable patients are those who cannot act on their own to protect themselves from threats to their health and dignity. Vulnerable patients are powerless.

Resources

Web site addresses are current as of this writing.

Codes of Ethical Conduct

American Medical Association Code of Medical Ethics

http://www.ama-assn.org/ama/pub/physician-resources/medical-ethics/code-medical-ethics.shtml

Canadian Medical Association Code of Medical Ethics
http://policybase.cma.ca/PolicyPDF/PD04-06.pdf

World Medical Association Code of Ethics
http://www.wma.net/en/30publications/10policies/c8/index.html

National Organizations for Guidance, Help, and Support

AARP (American Association of Retired Persons)
www.aarp.org

Alzheimer's Association
www.alz.org

Alzheimer Society of Canada
www.alzheimer.ca/english/index.php

American Academy of Hospice and Palliative Medicine
www.aahpm.org

American Heart Association
www.americanheart.org

American Lung Association
www.lungusa.org

Canadian Association of Retired Persons
www.carp.ca

Canadian Hospice Palliative Care Association
http://www.chpca.net/home.html

Canadian Lung Association
www.lung.ca/home-accueil_e.php

Heart and Stroke Foundation of Canada
www.heartandstroke.com/site/c.ikIQLcMWJtE/b.2796497/k.F922/Heart_Disease_Stroke_and_Healthy_Living.htm

FindLegalForms.com (living will forms for Canadian residents)
www.WillsandLegalForms.com (Canada)
www.findlegalforms.com/product/living-will-canada/

LawGuru Forms (living wills for United States residents)
http://g.forms.lawguru.com/living-wills_c.html

National Highway Traffic Safety Administration (older drivers program)
http://www.nhtsa.dot.gov/portal/site/nhtsa/menuitem.31176b9b03647a189ca8e410dba046a0/

Retirement Homes and related subjects
www.retirementhomes.com

Books

Beauchamp, TL, JF. Childress (eds.). *Principles of Biomedical Ethics*. New York: Oxford University Press, 2001.

Fries JF, Crapo LM. *Vitality and Aging*, W.H. Freeman and Company, 1981

Mindszenthy, BJ, Gordon M. *Parenting Your Parents: Support Strategies for Meeting the Challenge of Aging in America.* Toronto: Dundurn Press, 2006.

Olshansky J, *The Quest for Immortality*, W.W. Norton & Co, 2002

Pearson D, Shaw S. *Life Extension: A Practical and Scientific Approach*, Warner Books, New York, N.Y., 1982

Pipher M, *Another Country: Navigating the Emotional Terrain of Our Elders*, Riverhead Trade; 1st edition, 2000

Shem, S., *House of God*, Putnam, 1978, Dell, 1988, 2003

Singer, PA., Viens AM. (eds.). *The Cambridge Textbook of Bioethics.* Cambridge, N.Y; Cambridge University Press, 2008.

Walford R. *Maximum Life Span*, Maximum *Life Span.* New York: W.W. Norton & Co 1983, 1989, 2006

Walford R. *Beyond the 120 Year Diet: How to Double Your Vital Years,* Da Capo Press; Revised and Expanded edition, 2000

Edited Excerpts from the *Ethics at Baycrest Handbook: A Guide to Ethical Values and Commitments, Toronto, Ontario*, Third Edition (July 2006)

This handbook was developed at the Baycrest Geriatric Health Care System to assist family and staff members understand and integrate some of the important concepts of medical ethics into the decision-making process for patients, residents, and their families. The handbook was developed by the Baycrest Ethics Committee of which Dr. Michael Gordon is the chairperson.

Principles to Guide Decision Making

Clients (patients) and their families or substitute decision makers may be called on to make decisions, which have major consequences for themselves or others. Regardless of their magnitude, whether they involve day-to-day behavior or life and death situations, these decisions will have implications for the client's/patient's quality of life and perhaps for the lives of those around them. When challenged with difficult decisions, people find it helpful to have a framework to guide the decision-making process.

Care at any health care organization is provided in the context of a shared system of ethics and values that has been formulated by society as a whole, various legal and professional bodies, as well as our religious and cultural beliefs. A brief overview of the sources and specifics of the principles that guide clinical practice will provide a framework and context for the discussion of ethical issues that follows in this document.

The following are commonly accepted ethical principles that incorporate the shared values of our society and community and apply to the provision of care:

Sanctity of life—as part of Jewish religious principles (as well as those in other religions, cultures, and traditions), appreciation for the sanctity of life will influence decision-making when that value is important to the person and to those caring for the person.

Respect for persons—each person is unique with the right to have his or her unique needs addressed to the extent possible. The philosophy of client-centered care, espoused by many health care and long-term care facilities, expresses respect for persons.

Autonomy, Beneficence, Nonmaleficence, and Justice—important ethical principles are explained in the glossary of ethical terms.

Advance Care Planning

It is possible that at some point in the future you (client or patient) will become unable to make decisions for yourself. In the case of a condition like Alzheimer's disease, your ability to make your own decisions may decrease slowly over time. Alternatively, you may experience a sudden change in your decision-making ability due to situations such as a serious accident or stroke, or another medical condition that compromises intellectual function.

What is advance care planning?

You may choose to prepare for such a possibility by doing advance care planning. Advance care planning includes making decisions about the type of personal care, including health care, living arrangements, food, clothing, hygiene, and safety, that you want to receive in the future. This can be done by preparing a Power of Attorney for Personal Care in which you name a substitute decision maker.

A substitute decision maker is a person or persons who will make decisions on your behalf if you become incapable. Persons who are incapable are not able to understand the nature of treatment choices or appreciate the consequences of their decisions.

Why is advance care planning important?

Reasons for doing advance care planning include

- Ensuring that you receive the type of personal care you desire
- Promoting communication between you and your substitute decision maker(s), care providers, family, and friends
- Providing information that will help your substitute decision-maker(s) and health care providers make decisions about your personal care
- Reducing the burden of decision-making for your substitute decision-maker(s) and care providers

It should be understood that the preparation of a Power of Attorney for Personal Care (equivalent to the Health Care Surrogate or Health Care Power of Attorney in U.S. terminology) is **not** required in all jurisdictions but is often recommended to assure that those who make health care decisions are those who the person would have wanted to act on their behalf. In some jurisdictions there is a list by which people would become eligible (often family members) to make such decisions.

What is a Power of Attorney for Personal Care?

A Power of Attorney for Personal Care is a document in which you name a person or more than one person to be responsible for making personal decisions on your behalf should you become incapable. The person you name on the document is known as your Attorney for Personal Care. You can also provide written instructions about the type of personal care you do or do not want to receive should you become incapable at some point of time in the future. Decisions about life-sustaining treatments such as ventilators, intensive care, intravenous, and tube feeding may be included.

The Attorney(s) for Personal Care whom you name should be someone you trust, who knows you well, and is capable of making personal decisions on your behalf. It is important that you discuss your wishes with your Attorney for Personal Care. In general and it depends on the jurisdiction, the Power of Attorney for Personal Care only takes effect when you become incapable and hence are unable to make an informed decision.

Who will make decisions for me if I become incapable and have not prepared a Power of Attorney for Personal Care?

Depending on the jurisdiction, if you become incapable and do not have someone appointed to make decisions for you such as a guardian, Attorney for Personal Care, or a representative legally appointed by some authoritative body, there is usually a process by which such a person will be appointed legally to act on your behalf. In many jurisdictions there is a process by which various members of the family will be considered to be those who might act on your behalf—this can include the following in the order named but this might vary from one jurisdiction to another, and wherever you live, you should confirm what the order might be so that you can make sure you have either named someone specific or are comfortable with the normal sequence of those who can act in this capacity. An example of the sequence in the Province of Ontario is this:

1. Your spouse or partner
2. A child or parent
3. A brother or sister
4. Another relative
5. A suitable other unrelated person willing to act in this capacity

If there is more than one child, parent, or sibling, unless specifically named, all have equal status in substitute decision-making.

In other jurisdictions the sequence is usually comparable with the possibility of minor changes in sequence or priority

If I wish to do advance care planning, how should I proceed?

There are a number of people and resources available to assist you in this process. It is important that you discuss your health situation with your doctor and other members of the health care team. You may also wish to consult with a lawyer and/or a religious or spiritual leader. This will ensure that you are well informed and can make decisions that reflect your specific situation. It is also important to talk about advance care planning with your substitute decision maker(s), family, and friends.

What should I do if I already have a Power of Attorney for Personal Care?

If you have already prepared a Power of Attorney for Personal Care, it is important that your substitute decision maker(s) is aware of the document and familiar with its contents. You should also inform your doctor or another member of the health care team, so that they know whom to talk to when treatment decisions need to be made if you should become incapable. You should also provide a copy of the document to the institution in which you are being cared for especially if it is a long-term care facility or a nursing home.

Cardiopulmonary Resuscitation

Cardiopulmonary resuscitation (CPR) is a heroic form of medical treatment used when a person has suffered a cardiac and respiratory arrest. As this treatment is only potentially successful under limited and clearly defined circumstances, some organizations have developed protocols and medical practice guidelines for responding to cardiac arrest for clients residing in those facilities. The usual goals of the protocol and guidelines are these:

- To ensure that clients for whom CPR might be appropriate have the opportunity to make an informed decision regarding CPR or DNR, and
- to eliminate unnecessary and unwarranted CPR for clients who have died from a major medical condition or disease process and have not experienced a *true* cardiac or respiratory arrest, and for whom CPR would not be potentially successful.

The CPR/DNR protocol and guidelines have as their foundation the following principles:

- All clients/patients in long-term care facilities and nursing homes should be approached to discuss CPR/DNR as it relates to their health condition, unless they have indicated a desire not to have such a discussion. The content of any advance directives or living wills will be reviewed. When clients are not capable of participating in such discussions, inquiries will be made about wishes expressed when the client was capable.
- If a DNR order is not in place, CPR will be administered only if the client meets the medical indicators and guidelines for cardiac arrest. (See section below: What is a DNR order?)
- DNR orders will be reviewed on a regular basis and/or any other time at the request of the client or substitute decision maker.

CPR/DNR: A User's Guide for Clients and Family Members

Most people's understanding of cardiopulmonary resuscitation or CPR is based on what they have seen on television or at the movies. A person collapses from a heart attack and a crash cart, led by doctors and nurses, comes rushing down the hall to bring the victim back to life.

This popular image has led many people to believe that CPR is used to save someone from dying, or to bring a person who has died back to life. This is not a completely accurate picture of CPR.

What is CPR?

CPR is an emergency method of life saving under certain limited circumstances, usually an event which causes the heart to stop beating in a person who otherwise has normally working organs such as the heart, kidneys, liver, and brain. If these organs are significantly damaged, the body cannot sustain itself, and the heart stoppage is usually a result of the deterioration of the body in general.

CPR involves artificial respiration (breathing into the person's mouth or the use of a respirator bag) and external heart massage, usually after a sudden event such as a cardiac arrest, drowning, or high-voltage electric shock in a body that is otherwise reasonably healthy. If the heart is stopped for too long, permanent brain damage or death will occur, regardless of the cause of the heart stopping.

How effective is CPR?

CPR's effectiveness depends on the previous health of the person, the cause of the heart stoppage, and the speed with which CPR can be administered. CPR is most effective if begun within a few minutes after a cardiac arrest and if there is follow-up care in a hospital intensive care unit. It is most successful when the victim is a reasonably healthy person who has had a sudden loss of normal heart function. In these situations, attempting CPR may be worthwhile, with a survival rate ranging from 10 to 40 percent.

What is the role of CPR in long-term care/nursing home settings?

People who become patients and residents in long-term care settings such as nursing homes, homes for aged, and chronic care hospitals usually have many chronic health problems affecting many organs of the body including the heart, kidneys, liver, and brain. Research and experience have shown that CPR is unlikely to have a positive outcome for most of these individuals, especially when they are also very elderly. When someone with many chronic health problems has a cardiac arrest, it is usually not an isolated event nor is it likely to be reversible. The cardiac arrest is usually part of a complex process. Many parts of the body are already affected by disease, and a cardiac arrest is often the final step in a progressive and complex process of deterioration leading to death.

What are the chances of surviving cardiac arrest?

The odds of residents and patients in long-term care/nursing homes are low. Even under the best circumstances with the least compromised individuals, only 2 to 3 percent of people whose hearts stop unexpectedly will survive after receiving CPR. Based on studies of outcomes in long-term care facilities/nursing homes and other similar populations and, because of multiple pre-existing medical conditions, for the vast majority of clients residing in such facilities that are used for long-term care and not for short-term restorative care programs as is the case in some such facilities, the likelihood of surviving CPR is closer to zero.

Why not try CPR anyway?

If CPR were a simple, painless, and dignified procedure that was readily available, there would be no reason to recommend against using it in the long-term care setting. However, CPR requires intense treatment by doctors, nurses, and other staff members, and the procedure itself may cause painful damage to the chest wall, ribs, and internal organs.

CPR involves placing the person on a hard surface, either on a board if in bed or directly on the floor, pumping the chest vigorously and forcefully, and, at the same time, breathing for the person. A breathing tube may be inserted into the windpipe and oxygen delivered to assist in breathing. In many cases, an intravenous line must be quickly inserted to deliver medications, and it is often necessary to apply a number of electrical shocks to the heart through paddles placed on the chest.

Some people residing in a long-term care setting respond at first to the CPR treatment. It is then usually necessary to transfer them to an intensive care unit at an acute care hospital to be maintained on a respirator. However, the vast majority of people who survive at first in these circumstances die within a few hours or days.

Why is this information important?

When clients are admitted to long-term care facilities/nursing homes, the staff usually wants to do everything humanly possible to make them comfortable and maximize their ability to take part in activities and enjoy life. However, it is usually felt by the staff that they have a duty to make sure that clients and families are made aware of the facts about the CPR procedure and its outcome in this population, before discussions are held about the possibility of a DNR (Do Not Resuscitate) order.

What is a DNR order?

A DNR order will protect the person from unnecessary attempts at CPR, which will offer virtually no medical benefit. When a person has agreed to a DNR order, this order is written into the health care record (the chart) by the physician. It tells the medical and nursing staff that, in the event of disorder affecting the heart such as a heart attack or other cause of cardiac arrest, certain resuscitative procedures are not to be started. If there is no DNR order, CPR will only be tried if the person has had a cardiac arrest in circumstances in which it is medically indicated: the event is witnessed (observed) by a health care provider and the person is not suffering from an illness which has been shown to negate any of the potential benefits of CPR. The vast majority of our clientele at long-term care facilities and nursing homes suffer from such illnesses. Even in the absence of a DNR, the staff is not obliged to undertake CPR unless the event is witnessed and the person is not suffering from a condition (such as an acute infection, heart failure, impaired kidney function, a recent stroke) that would make the exercise futile in terms of possible success.

A DNR order applies only to the process of CPR and not to any other medical treatments. All other treatments can be considered and decisions about them will be made as usual, based on the person's needs and interests and potential benefits. In general, the practice in long-term care facilities and nursing homes should be that all clients/patients, regardless of a DNR order, will receive the treatment and care necessary to ensure their maximum functioning and comfort.

Reference: Gordon, M. CPR in Long-Term Care: Mythical Benefits or Necessary Ritual? *Annals of Long-Term Care,* Volume 11, April 2003.

To Transfer and/or to Treat

As in any multi-level care system, not all forms of acute medical treatment and symptom management are available in all locations within most long-term care facilities/nursing homes. In situations in which the client's/patients' condition could be improved by treatments available elsewhere, most long-term care facilities/nursing homes will offer transfer to an acute care hospital.

In nonemergency situations, the decision to transfer and the alternative courses of treatment and expected outcomes will be discussed with the client or substitute decision maker in advance. In emergency situations, the decision to transfer and/or to treat will be based on the known wishes of the client or substitute decision maker and the attending physician's assessment of the situation.

A decision not to treat or not to transfer to an acute care facility may be appropriate in some cases, especially when a client is terminally ill. In such situations, most long-term care facilities/nursing homes will endeavor to cooperate with the client's or substitute decision maker's choice and provide appropriate treatment and care in place, or transfer the person to a local Palliative Care or Hospice Unit if one exists external to the facility or within such a unit if it exists within the facility.

Nutrition and Hydration

Some long-term care/nursing home facilities provide programs of eating assistance strategies. The purpose of these programs is to maintain clients'/patients' abilities to eat for as long as possible. The programs usually aim to prevent the development of excess disability in eating and to enable clients to feed themselves to the extent possible. Clients/patients with eating difficulties are generally assessed in a variety of ways including observing eating habits, exploring preferences and physical limitations, conducting swallowing studies, and measuring nutritional intake. Based on the assessment, appropriate foods and food textures are usually offered and an individualized care plan is developed. These plans usually detail a program for maximizing independence in eating while providing the required assistance through appropriate utensils, visual and other sensory cues, and feeding when necessary. The extent and nature of such programs depends on the jurisdiction and the mandate or requirements of long-term care/nursing home facilities and may vary widely.

In general, in situations when a thorough evaluation shows that a client/patient cannot swallow or eat in a manner adequate to maintain sufficient nutrition, or that feeding by mouth constitutes a danger, other appropriate feeding methods may be proposed to provide liquid food on a continuous basis. Options include temporary measures such as a tube inserted through a vein (intravenous) or below the skin for the purpose of hydration (hypodermoclysis). More permanent approaches include a tube through the nose (nasogastric), or directly into the stomach (gastrostomy). Only the latter process is generally used for long periods, as a tube through the nose is generally uncomfortable on a long-term basis. Organizations must recognize the right of clients/patients with the capacity to make decisions, or substitute decision makers of those clients who are not capable who have knowledge of the person's wishes, to refuse the insertion of feeding or intravenous devices. Such clients residing in Baycrest will continue to be offered food and liquids by mouth. Long-term care facilities/nursing homes are generally expected by law to support an approach to care that provides nutrition and hydration in keeping with the individual client's/patient's right to choose the method of nutrition or refuse any artificial method of nutrition and hydration.

Decisions about inserting feeding, intravenous, or subcutaneous devices are made on an individual basis in the context of the individual's condition and prognosis. Clients/patients and substitute decision makers are encouraged to consult with their care team, spiritual leader, family members, or other significant persons before making a decision. The advantages of tube feeding, including maintaining nutrition and hydration and potentially prolonging life, must be weighed against the disadvantages which may include physical discomfort during placement and complications while the tube is in place. When the client is not competent to make the decision, all efforts will be made to learn what the client/patient would have wanted, given the client's/patient's condition and prognosis, and the benefits and burdens of the treatment.

When the views of the client residing in a long-term care/nursing home cannot be determined and the substitute decision maker agrees, consideration will be given to a trial of tube feeding. Such a trial may be seen as a step that would give the substitute decision makers and the clinical team more time to reflect and to observe the client's/patient's response, both clinically and behaviorally. At the conclusion of the pre-specified period of time (for example, one or two months), the team, in consultation with the family or significant others, may re-evaluate and decide whether or not tube feeding should be extended or terminated, based on whether the goals of the process were or were not achieved. As in all situations in which clients/patients resist feeding, the causes of any resistance to tube feeding should be thoroughly explored.

The ethical principles used in nutrition/hydration decisions are enumerated below:

Decisions regarding tube feeding are often highly emotional and may involve resolving conflicting beliefs and values. The ethical principles of Respect for Persons, Autonomy, and Beneficence are some that might be considered during the deliberations and discussion among those who ultimately will make the necessary decisions. These principles may at times be in conflict with each other. In such cases a thoughtful ethical discussion involving the team and the patient/family/substitute decision maker (SDM) should take place to attempt to resolve dilemmas. The organization's ethicist or members of the clinical ethics committee if these bodies and structures exist in the institution are potential resources that may also be included in the discussions.

Some of the issues to be considered during the discussion are these:

Respect for Individuals

- Valuing the unique quality of each patient's needs
- Treating the client in a dignified manner
- Respecting family, cultural, and religious beliefs, and the meanings associated with eating
- Encouraging options that are in the patient's best interest

Autonomy

- Respecting the client's right to make informed choices about treatment options. For example, a patient might choose to have a feeding tube inserted and may later change his/her mind and wish it to be removed. The client or SDM's decision must be respected.
- When the patient is deemed incompetent to make this decision, the SDM will decide among treatment options according to the patient's previously stated competent wishes; when that knowledge is absent, currently made decisions are to be in accordance with the best interests of the patient. Even when the client is deemed incompetent, the family and team members must consider the client's behavioral and emotional responses to the treatment offered when assessing the benefits and burdens of continuing it.

Beneficence

- Promoting client's welfare/best interest
- Maximizing safety (for example, by avoiding aspiration)
- Maximizing pleasure (for example, joy related to tasting of food, or being fed by a loved one)
- Maximizing comfort
- Increasing quality of life
- Prolonging life

Nonmaleficence

- Avoiding risks of oral feeding when swallowing problems exist
- Avoiding the results of chronic malnutrition such as skin breakdown if adequate nutrition cannot be taken by mouth

About the Author

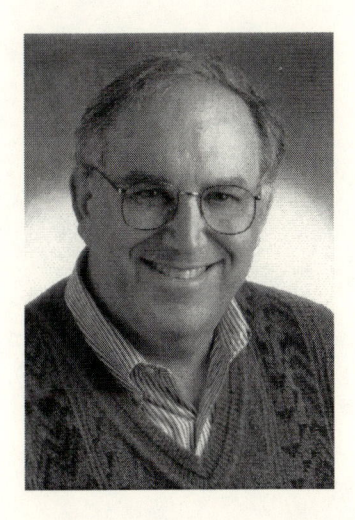

As the holder of Canada's first certificate as a specialist in Geriatric Medicine, issued in 1981, **Dr. Michael Gordon** has been at the forefront of the establishment and growth of this medical specialty in Canada, and of the resulting advances in geriatric care provision. His interest in the ethical aspects of caring for the elderly grew out of his career-long experience with families struggling to make difficult decisions on behalf of their loved ones. Looking for answers, a post-graduate degree in Ethics helped to propel Dr. Gordon into not only the practice of medical ethics but also into writing and teaching medical students and professionals, as well as the lay public, about the challenging and often heart-wrenching decisions that sometimes have to be made.

Moments that Matter was written for family members faced with difficult decisions in providing care for a loved one. The goal of the book is to provide those surrogate decision-makers with the confidence that they have done everything possible to achieve the wishes of their loved ones in a way that reflects personal values and family principles.

Index

A

acute care systems
  hospitals as, 97–98
  treatment decisions in, 98–106
admission
advance care planning, 161–170
  about, 161–163
  AHN, 168–170 (See also AHN (artificial nutrition and hydration))
  autonomy, 170 (See also autonomy)
  beneficence, 170 (See also beneficence)
  CPR and DNR, 163–167 (See also CPR (Cardiopulmonary Resuscitation); DNR (do not resuscitate) orders)
  definition of, 151
  nonmaleficence (See nonmaleficence (avoidance of harm))
  nonmaleficence (avoidance of harm), 170
  respecting others, 170
  transferring treatment, 167–168
advance directives (living wills), 47–48, 111, 128–131, 151
age-based medical care, challenges of, 55–59
ageism, 56–58
AgeLab, Massachusetts Institute of Technology's, 32
aging, nature of, 1–5
aging family members, 6–11, 45–48
  See also parents, aging
aging population, needs of, 1, 19
AHN (artificial nutrition and hydration), 62, 80, 81–82, 84–85, 91, 151, 168–169
Alzheimer's disease
  advance care planning and, 161
  CPR and, 110
  driving with, 32–35, 36
  ethics of doing the right thing and, 13
  rates of, 1
  resources for, 157
  sex and romance decisions and, 37, 39–40
  truth-telling in, 49–52
  See also dementia
Alzheimer's Disease and Memory Disorders Center (Rhode Island), 32
American Lung Association, 4
amputations, 66–68
Annals of Internal Medicine, "Controlling Death" (Perkins), 130
Annals of Long-Term Care, "CPR in Long-Term Care" (Gordon), 167
Another Country (Pipher), 40, 159

anti-aging, promotion of, 21, 22–23
"Anti-Aging Medicine" (Journals of Gerontology), 21
antibiotics, 20, 70, 74–75, 85, 93, 95
arthritis, 4
artificial nutrition and hydration (AHN), 62, 80, 81–82, 84–85, 91, 151, 168–169
autonomy, 170
   artificial nutrition and hydration (AHN) and, 169
   in choosing long-term care facilities, 121
   consent to treatment and, 98–99
   decision-making and, 8, 10, 15, 59
   declining therapy as part of, 70, 138
   definition of, 151
   informed decisions and, 82–83, 87, 89
   surrogate decision-making and, 46
   truth-telling and, 51
   vaccinations and, mandatory, 147
Away from Her (movie), 39

B

balancing, 99
   benefits and harms, 49–54
   decision-making, 17
   ethical principles, 82–83, 99
   giving and receiving, 92–96
   and principlist approach to ethics, 17
   when goals conflict, 60–62
Baycrest Handbook
   advance care planning, 161–163
   autonomy, 170
   beneficence, 170

CPR (Cardiopulmonary Resuscitation), 163–167
DNR (do not resuscitate) orders, 164–167
nonmaleficence, 170
nutrition and hydration, 168–169
principles to guide decision-making, 160
respect for others, 170
transfer and/or to treat patients, 167–168
Beauchamp, TL, Principles of Biomedical Ethics, 158
bed blocking, 55
beneficence, 170
   artificial nutrition and hydration (AHN) and, 169
   definition of, 151
   family member roles and, 15
   health care professionals and, 99
   health care professionals with, 144
   informed decisions and, 82, 84, 89
   nonmaleficence linked to, 153
   priciplism and, 154
best interest standard, definition of, 152
best interterst decision, 84
Beyond the 120-Year Diet (Walford), 22, 159
Bush, Jeb, 63

C

The Cambridge Textbook of Bioethics (Singer &Viens), 159
Canadian Lung Association, 4
Canadian Medical Association
   on euthanasia and withdrawal of treatment, 82

resources for Code of Medical
Ethics, 157
cancer, 13, 51–53, 124
capable, legal concept, 152
cardiac arrest, 92, 96, 109–112,
164, 165–166, 167
Cardiopulmonary Resuscitation See
CPR
caregivers, veracity and, 155
caregiving decisions
challenging, many players in,
63–65
ethical framework of, 2
Catholicism, 9, 47, 64, 68–70, 134
chemotherapy, 51, 53, 128, 153
Childress, JF, Principles of
Biomedical Ethics, 158
choices, personal, 8, 70, 147, 151
See also informed consent
Christie, Julie, 39
chronic care hospitals, 66, 68, 73,
165
code of ethical conduct, resources
for, 157
code of ethics, professional,
definition of, 154
codes of conduct, ethical framework,
144
cognitive impairment, 29, 32–33,
38, 41, 85, 99, 122–123
Cole, Thomas R., 40
communication
about CPR, 111
about difficult decisions, 10–11,
125
about palliative care, 136, 137
end of life process, during, 127–
128
between families and health care
staff, 148–149
truth-telling in concept of, 51

of values, 73
competent, legal concept, definition
of, 152
compromises, 61, 80, 91, 147, 149,
152, 161
Connor, Stephen, 141
consent to treatment, 98–100
continuing care units, 92, 93
"Controlling Death" (Perkins), 130
Cox, Lynne, 23
CPR (Cardiopulmonary
Resuscitation), 95–96, 107–113,
138, 152, 163–167
"CPR in Long-Term Care"
(Gordon), 167
CPR procedure, 166
Crapo, LM, Vitality and Aging, 22,
24, 158
Cruzan, Nancy, 134
cultural views, in decision-making,
71

D

death See end-of-life
decision-making
ageism in, 56–58
AHN (artificial nutrition and
hydration) and, 80–82, 84–85,
91, 151, 168–169
balance in, 17
based on relationships, 8
conflicts in, 60–62, 103–105,
148–149
disagreeing with health care
professionals, 89–91, 144
end-of-life, 76–77
ethical considerations for, 7–8, 10
interpreting decisions to health
care professionals, 71
religious and cultural views of, 71

See also substitute decision
   makers; surrogate decision
   makers
dementia
   ageism and, 57
   care for, 26
   decision-making for, 6–9, 123
   ethics of doing the right thing
      and, 9
   strain on family members and, 6,
      8
   See also Alzheimer's disease
dementia patients, driving privileges
   and, 32
Department of Motor Vehicles
   (United States), driving
   assessments, 33
diabetes, 35, 66, 72, 98, 110
dialysis, 17–18, 22, 47, 73, 103,
   153
diets, low calorie, 22
dignified death, 70, 112
distributive justice (fairness), 16, 24,
   56, 95, 152, 153
 See also justice
DNR (do not resuscitate) orders,
   108, 109–110, 111–112, 113,
   164, 166–167
drinking, and feeding
   AHN (artificial nutrition and
      hydration) as, 80, 81–82,
      84–85, 91, 151, 168–169
   basic need for, 78–79, 81–82
   ethical dilemmas around, 90–91
   feeding by mouth, 86–89
   meaning of, 79–81
DriveAble (Canada), 33
driving privileges, losing, 27, 28, 28,
   30–34
drugs See medications
duties, professional, 154

duty
   to avoid causing harm, 15-16
   to be truthful, 51
   of care, professional, 145, 148
   definition of, 152
   parental, 63
   to report, as physicians, 33
   to support decisions, 70, 71

E

eating, and drinking See feeding,
   and drinking
Ecclesiastes, 25
emergency room (ER), 97, 99, 101,
   111
end-of-life
   dignified death at, 70, 112
   food and drink during, 62, 79,
      80, 81
   life extension at, 19–25
   medical care decisions, 59, 96,
      117, 131–135, 144
   palliative care at, 136–142
   process, 127–128
   quality of life decisions, 71, 76–77
   rituals and practices, 126–127
   situations, 9, 13–15, 124
   See also living wills (advance
      directives)
ethical challenges, xi, xii, 8, 25, 80,
   89–91, 92, 146
ethical concepts, applying, 12–14
ethical dilemmas, 90, 152
ethical frameworks
   of decision-making, 2, 8–9
   for determining sexual and
      romance relationships, 36–37
   of practice, Codes of Conduct,
      144
ethical principles

176

autonomy (See autonomy)
beneficence (See beneficence)
justice, 16, 17, 24, 40, 56, 95, 152, 153, 154
nonmaleficence (avoidance of harm), 15–16, 89, 99, 153, 154, 160, 170
related to long-term care facilities, 114
religious and cultural view translated into, 71

ethicists
definition of, 152
involvement for end-of-life decisions, 130, 131, 133
involvement in choice if treatment, 95, 125
involvement in working through issues, 64
and surrogate decision maker, 43–44, 48

ethics
of ageism, 56
concepts and meaningful action of, 12–14
meaning of, 15–16
of medical treatment withdrawal, 82
narrative, 17–19

ethics committees
definition of, 153
involvement for end-of-life decisions, 131, 133
involvement in working through issues, 64, 125

euthanasia
definition of, 153
passive, 154
use of drugs to hasten death vs., 138, 140

vs. withdrawal of treatment, 82, 132
exercising, older people and, 4

F

family dynamics, 7–9, 17
family structure, maintaining, 6
feeding, and drinking
AHN (artificial nutrition and hydration) as, 62, 80, 81–82, 84–85, 91, 151, 168–169
basic need for, 78–79, 81–82
ethical dilemmas around, 90–91
feeding by mouth, 86–89
meaning of, 79–81
flu shots, 145–147
Fries, JF, Vitality and Aging, 22, 24, 158
funerals, prearranging, 127–128

G

geriatric assessments, 9–11
geriatrics, 55, 57–58
glossary of ethical terms, 151–155
goals
in complex situations, 95–96
conflict of, 60–62, 148–149
of palliative care, 136, 138, 140, 142
Gordon, Michael
"CPR in Long-Term Care", 167
Parenting Your Parents, 159
guide to ethical values See Baycrest Handbook
guilt, 9–11, 65, 132
Gulliver's Travels (Swift), 23

H

H1N1 (swine flu), 146–147

Harvard Medical School Letter, 22
health care changes, making, 3–4
health care field, multicultural environments and, 71
Health Care Power of Attorney
  advance care planning and, 151
  definition of, 154
health care professionals
  ethical perspective of, 143–149
  transfer and/or treat, 167–168
health care system
  aging and, nature of, 1–5
  using, 4–5
heart attacks, 4, 20, 57, 92, 100–101, 167
heart disease, 3–4, 35, 110, 158
heart massage, external, 165
Hendry, Joene, 32
heroic measures, 28, 75, 129
Holocaust, 17, 18
home care agencies, 11
hospice, 140, 141, 142, 157, 158, 168
hospitals
  as acute care systems, 97–98
  bed blocking in, 55
  chronic care, 66, 68, 73, 165
  consent to treatment in, 98–100
  continuing care units, 92, 93
  CPR situations in, 109
  Medicare payment for adverse outcomes in, 5
House of God (Shem), 55, 159
hydration, artificial, 62, 151

I

influenza, 146–147
informed consent, 82–83, 87, 89, 153
Institute of Medicine, "Retooling for an Aging America," 57–58
Internet Web sites, 33, 157–158
"Is It Ever Too Late For Love and Romance" (Medical Post), 39

J

Journal of Pain and Symptom Management, use of opiates, 141
Journals of Gerontology, "Anti-Aging Medicine," 21
Judaism, 22, 66–67, 133–134, 160
judgment, substituted, 155
justice, 16, 17, 24, 40, 56, 95, 152, 153, 154

K

Kantian ethics, 152

L

Leipzig, Rosanne M., 57
license, lose of driver's, 30–34
life expectancy, 14, 19–20, 22–25, 40
life extension, 19–25
Life Extension (Pearson and Shaw), 22, 159
life-sustaining treatments, definition of, 153
living wills (advance directives), 47, 48, 111, 128–131
  definition of, 151
long-term care facilities (nursing home care)
  care in, 55, 123–125
  CPR in, 167
  deciding on, 117–123
  desperation and, sense of, 80
  meaning of term, 114

navigating the system in, 115–116
    See also nursing homes
"Love in the Time of Dementia" (Zernike), 39–40

M

Massachusetts Institute of Technology's AgeLab, 32
Maximum Life Span (Walford), 22, 159
medical ethics See ethical principles
Medical Post, Canada (magazine), "Is It Ever Too Late For Love and Romance," 39
Medicare, 5, 57–58
medications
    and Alzheimer's disease, 51
    for mental impairment, 28
    morphine, use of, 138–139, 141
    opiates, use of, 137, 139–141
    to prolong life, 22–23
    use in decision-making, 122
Mindszenthy, BJ, Parenting Your Parents, 159
morphine, use of, 138–139, 141
Muslims, 134
myths, about aging, 2–4

N

narrative ethics, 17–19
National Highway Traffic Safety Administration, older drivers program, 33
National Hospice and Palliative Care Organization, on use of opiates, 141
national organizations for guidance, resources for, 157–158
Nature (journal), 22

neurological issues, 33, 62, 68, 73, 80
New England Journal of Medicine, CPR survival rates, 107
New York Times
    "Love in the Time of Dementia" (Zernike), 39–40
    "The Patients Doctors Don't Know", 57
nonmaleficence (avoidance of harm), 15–16, 89, 99, 153, 154, 160, 170
nurses
nursing home care (long-term care), 55
    care in, 123–125
    deciding on, 117–123
    meaning of term, 114
    navigating the system in, 115–116
nursing homes
    CPR situations in, 109–111
    DNR orders in, 112
    sex and romance in, 35–39
nursing units, skilled, 92, 93
nutrition, artificial, 62, 80–82, 84–85, 91, 151

O

O'Connor, Sandra Day, 39–40
Olshansky, Jay, 25
    The Quest for Immortality, 23, 159
opiates, use of, 137, 139–141
Ott, Brian R., 32

P

pain management, 13, 15–16, 137–141
palliative care

choosing, 103–104, 124, 127, 136–142, 168
  definition of, 153–154
  resources for, 158
Parenting Your Parents (Mindszenthy & Gordon), 159
parents, aging
  activities and, 30–34
  caring for, 24–30, 58–59
  decision-making for, 103–105
  goal conflicts for, 60–62
  living will with, 111
  long-term care facilities (nursing home care) and (See long-term care facilities (nursing home care))
  sex and romance for, 34–41
  surrogate decision makers for, 42–48
  wishes of, knowing, 59
  See also aging family members
Parkinson's disease, 4, 60, 72
passive euthanasia, definition of, 154
patients
  geriatric, 57–58
  health care professional conflicts with, 148–149
  truth-telling with, 51, 52
  vulnerable, 155
"The Patients Doctors Don't Know" (New York Times), 57
Pearson, D., Life Extension, 22, 159
Perkins, Henry S., "Controlling Death", 130
persistent vegetative state, 63–64
  See also vegetative state
personal choices, 8, 70, 147, 151
  See also informed consent
personal values, 47, 69, 77, 85, 90
physician-assisted suicide, 138
  See also euthanasia
Pinsent, Gordon, 39
Pipher, M., Another Country, 40, 159
pneumonia, 29, 69, 84, 86–88, 93–94, 98
Polley, Sarah, 39
Power of Attorney for Personal Care
  advance care planning and, 151, 161–163
  definition of, 154
Principles of Biomedical Ethics (Beauchamp & Childress), 158
principles of contemporary medical ethics, 16
  See also ethical principles
principlism, definition of, 154
principlist approach to ethics, 17
  See also ethical principles
procedural justice, definition of, 153
  See also justice
professional code of ethics, 154
professional values (duties), definition of, 154

Q

quality of life
  AHN (artificial nutrition and hydration) and, 80 (See also artificial nutrition and hydration (AHN))
  definition of, 155
  discontinuing treatment and, 103
  religious views of, 66–71, 134
  secular views of, 71–77
Quinlan, Karen, 134

R

relationships, decision-making based on, 8

respirators, 69, 99, 102, 104–105, 132, 143, 155
resuscitation, 107–109, 112, 167
retirement homes, 114–116, 120–121
  See also long-term care facilities (nursing home care)
"Retooling for an Aging America" (Institute of Medicine), 57–58
"right to life," decisions, 64
romance and sex
  in nursing homes, 35–39
  for older people, 34–35

S

safety issues
  driving as, 30–34
  wandering as, 122
sanctity of life, 68–69, 132, 134, 155, 160
"sandwich" generation, 24
SARS, 2003 (Ontario), 145–147
Schiavo, Terri, 63–64
Schiavo case, 129, 134
sex and romance
  in nursing homes, 35–39
  for older people, 34–35
Shaw, S., Life Extension, 22, 159
Shem, Samuel, House of God, 55, 159
Singer, PA, The Cambridge Textbook of Bioethics, 159
skilled nursing units, 92, 93
smoking, cessation of, 3–4
societal resources, use of, 3
"squaring the curve," 24
stereotypes, 40–41
strokes, 26, 66, 80–81, 90, 105, 158, 167
Strong, Randy, 22

substitute decision makers, 83, 85, 151, 160–161, 163–164, 167–169
  See also surrogate decision makers
substituted judgment, definition of, 155
suicide See euthanasia
surrogate decision makers
  artificial nutrition and hydration (AHN) and, 81 (See also artificial nutrition and hydration (AHN))
  consent to treatment and, 99, 138–139
  definition of, 155
  ethical and legal responsibilities for, 8–9, 87–88, 89–90
  individuals and, 42–48
  living wills helping, 130
  long-term care facilities assessment, 122, 123
  making choices of treatment, 95–96
  role of, 37, 45, 46
  value systems, understanding, 76
  See also decision-making; substitute decision makers
Swift, Jonathan, Gulliver's Travels, 23
Swine flu (H1N1), 146–147
symptom management, 14, 124, 129, 136, 138, 141, 167

T

treatment decisions, 98–106, 131–135
truth-telling, 49–54

U

U.S. Supreme Court cases, on stopping treatment, 134, 143–144

V

vaccinations, 145–148
values
   personal, 47, 69, 77, 85, 90
   professional, definition of, 154
vegetative state, 63–64, 69–70
ventilators, 104–105, 131, 153, 154, 155, 162
veracity, definition of, 155
Viens AM, The Cambridge Textbook of Bioethics, 159
Vitality and Aging (Fries and Crapo), 22, 24, 158
vulnerable patients (person), definition of, 155

W

Walford, R.
   Beyond the 120-Year Diet, 22, 159
   Maximum Life Span, 22, 159
Web sites, 33, 157–158

Z

Zernike, Kate, "Love in the Time of Dementia" (New York Times), 39